What others

"The book chapters are clear accounts/ "case" descriptions of the culture, health care, and living conditions of people living in countries where the real-life stories occurred. Writing the book [based on many years of your work with the medical missions] indeed reflects a personal journey."

Phoebe D. Williams, PhD, RN, FAAN

"All mothers desire to have a healthy baby, a truism embraced within one's heart and soul as pregnancy is recognized. Trust, cultural beliefs, and spirituality surrounding birth are uniquely captured in the book, All Babies are Born. Stories from a global context include the joy and challenges of American midwives supporting women giving birth in under resourced countries. Particular focus guides the reader in experiences of one midwife's journey within herself, birthing women, and God. Through descriptive scenes, voices of women, and Scripture, one notes the profound call for global recognition of the unnecessary and devastating losses of human life. Voices rarely heard by those who do not suffer similar geographic disparities. This book will move you to action."

Ginger Breedlove, PhD, CNM, ARNP, FACNM

"Cathy Gordon, midwife and missionary lifts up the essence of global birth disparities viewed through a Christian lens. As she describes her journeys into sweltering rain forest and barren institutional hospitals, we are tucked inside her pocket, meeting laboring mothers through her eyes. I laughed with her during moments of absurdity and sighed out loud at her frustration of not being able to fully practice her craft in absence of simple supplies. It is my deepest hope that American mothers read this book. We will cry, we will get mad, and then, we will act.

Kendra Wyatt, Co-Founder New Birth Company L3C

"Catherine Gordon's knowledge, skill and passion for nurse midwifery are personified in this book which tells the story of her personal journey to assist women through childbirth. She shares her stories, secrets, faith, compassion, and wisdom as she travels through nine countries to assist vulnerable populations bring new life into the world. Many of the women and families in these exemplars bring with them significant psychosocial, cultural and environmental issues that put them at increased risk for poor obstetric outcomes. This book brings to the forefront the true value of the midwifery model of care."

Helen R. Connors, PhD, RN, FAAN

All Babies are Born

*a midwifery journey
to the ends of the earth*

Catherine Gordon

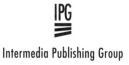

Intermedia Publishing Group

All Babies are Born

Published by:
Intermedia Publishing Group, Inc.
P.O. Box 2825
Peoria, Arizona 85380
www.intermediapub.com

ISBN 978-1-935906-56-8

Dedication

This is book is written for families who have experienced birth. It is dedicated to women who have experienced birth in developing countries. It is also dedicated to the birth attendants, who aid women in the most difficult setting while women are giving birth with limited medications and supplies. May God continue to bless their hands, and the women they serve.

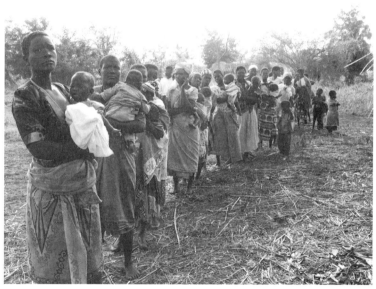

These woman and babies are waiting in line to see a health care provider. We were their only health care provider.

He Carried Her Home

A small wooden building that housed a three-room clinic was our new home. Rustic, modest and remote, this setting was our place of rest after our long journey to the village of Francis Sirpi, Nicaragua. Unfortunately, we had no running water or electricity. We stumbled across each other in search of a place to lay our weary bodies.

Our team of seven emergency department staff, traveled for hours by plane to Managua, then chartered a flight into the remote village. Our goal was to offer health care to those in need at a small rural health clinic. Homeland to the Miskito Indians, Nicaragua is known as one of the most remote and poorly developed countries of the Western hemisphere. Poverty is rampant in the sparsely populated western and southern areas of the country, once savagely reduced in size due to government unrest and war.

"This is what I call camping" said one of my long-time friends and a nurse as she dozed off to sleep mumbling something about her version of camping being more like a Motel six.

Night stars illuminated the sky while kerosene lanterns provided a source of light so we could safely move about the camp. Rest was welcome after carrying over 100 pounds of medical supplies and medicines. Looking up from my wooden bunk, I could see the vast heavens peering through cracks in the planks that made up the roof. The magnitude of stars covered the sky from east to west. The expanse of the Milky Way and cascading stars lured me into a deep, restful sleep.

Our first day of camp was one that would be a life changing adventure for our small team . We planned to hike to a remote area, untouched by non-traditional healthcare providers like us. Nationals typically sought health care from the local witch doctor and used his remedies for their ailments. Most had never seen or considered treatment from a medical doctor or health care provider. With this in mind, we were unsure whether or not we would have any willing patients.

We gathered supplies, medicines, and remedies for the day and loaded them into the back of a pick-up truck. Our guide, a Nicaraguan national and native Miskito Indian, led the way by pointing and jabbering his directions. Road conditions were typical of pastures in Kansas with rocks, dirt clods and no definite markers except an occasional cattle trail. Unfortunately, there were no cattle paths, paved, or asphalted roads here. The locals sauntered along the pathway.

Onward ho, I thought, as I sat in the back of the truck, jostling from side to side.

The truck stopped abruptly. The small single bridge over a gently flowing river was missing, washed out by torrential rains. No road crews or heavy equipment were available to repair the bridge, so the villagers on the other side were captive to failing governmental infrastructures. We were also separated from the village. The only way to get there was to lift our backpacks and begin the five-mile hike first around the river and then to the village.

Bearing my backpack, water bottle, and camera, I soon began the trek. Antibiotics, pain relievers, vitamins and various medical supplies weighed over fifty pounds each. The shoulder straps, worn from years of use, seemed to cut into my flesh. We tromped across the countryside amidst the high humidity and soaring heat. Parched with thirst, I drank often from my water bottle. My backpack seemed to get heavier and heavier. Just as we arrived at the village, I finished my water. I knew God would supply our needs, so I stopped to pray with our friends for relief from the heat and the thirst that overwhelmed us.

Curious villagers, some of whom hid in their small wooden homes, peeked at us. Other brave souls ventured out to meet us. I found a log to sit on and rested my weakened body.

The village leader approached with the usual greeting of the Miskito Indians. The long hellos and greetings of one's family to another is common and must not be overlooked. It is respectful to always greet first, then inquire about health and well-being before the inquiry of "Why are you here?"

Our guide shared with the leader that we had come to impart a blessing on his village —to offer health care, freely, just as Christ had freely given His gift of salvation to us. The village leader was happy to receive us, and to aide us in fulfilling our purpose. He directed us to a building where we could hold the clinic.

Composed of large wood planks, pillars held up the rough ceiling. With no walls, the building resembled Woodstock in Virginia with an open amphitheater of sorts and a platform for performing arts. Briefly, I wondered if they had any performing arts here, but decided— probably not.

Our group gathered logs for seating, made tables for consultations and laid cloths on the ground for exam areas. The makeshift clinic took shape rapidly and each of us set our stations strategically apart so we could perform exams and maintain a slight degree of privacy. The village dwellers came, one by one, then in family groups. We treated a variety of maladies such as malaria, chagas, scleroderma, various infections, multiple pains and much more. Every individual and family received antiparasititics treatment and vitamins. We performed consultations, gave medications, and expected no payment for our services or medications. God had freely given to us; therefore, we freely gave to His Nicaraguan people.

Working for over four hours in the intense heat, after hiking five miles, my thirst became a constant reminder of the heat. The shade helped cool our dehydrated bodies. Midday, my head began to pound and I wondered if I could make the trek back to camp. I felt like I was suffering the beginnings of heat exhaustion. Our team leader, a savvy nurse, noted our need for water. She called on the village dwellers and asked them to go find coconuts.

The men quickly mobilized and ascended the tall palm trees, cutting down large coconuts with their machetes. Within minutes, about thirty coconuts came to our rescue, much more than we needed. Just as quickly as they retrieved the coconuts, the men helped us open them. They were masters of this sport. The quenching liquid of the coconuts immediately satisfied our thirst. Amazingly, we each drank two. We topped off our water bottles with the remaining coconut milk. I felt so refreshed and invigorated; I wondered if the Gatorade people knew about these coconuts. We were so grateful. Despite our lack of preparation,

God had taken care of our need. That was by far the best coconut I have ever had.

Our clinic continued until mid-afternoon. Darkness loomed on the horizon, as well as hungry mosquitoes. After packing up our remaining supplies, we began the five-mile trek back to our truck. My backpack, now reduced of its weight, seemed much easier to carry. The coconut milk gave us energy and helped us get back quicker. We arrived at the truck; our bodies dehydrated yet our spirits exhilarated, as the sun quickly set.

Thirsty and famished again, I could do nothing more than make jokes about my favorite foods and the quenching drinks back home. Everyone laughed. While waiting on our driver, we noticed a tree full of ripe fruit. I ran across the road and reached for the fruit.

Our Indian companion warned me, "The fruit is poison. You should not eat of it." He described a wrenching and painful death, according to the words of the trusted witch doctor.

I stopped picking fruit, but my American mindset took over. *What? Why can't we eat this fruit when it looks good?*

I remembered the Old Testament story as I reflected on the forbidden fruit in the Garden of Eden. I wasn't taking this fruit to gain wisdom, but to satisfy my thirst. I wondered if the words of our guide were true. Could this be forbidden fruit?

My strong will won. With the encouragement of our American team, I reached for one of the largest fruit that must have weighed about five pounds. I smelled the fruit, wondering if Nicaraguan poison smelled a certain way. The fruit seemed normal. Reaching for several, I tossed one to each of my companions. Without a care in the world, I grasped the large yellow fruit, peeled it and indulged in the juicy flavor. It was so sweet, and the juice ran down my chin and dripped to the ground. I grabbed more fruit for our team and our Indian companions then tossed my harvest into the back of our truck.

The Indians soon realized this fruit was good to eat and they too joined in our feast. As we drove back to camp, we learned that years of war had taken a large percentage of the Indian population. Many orphans grew up thinking this fruit was forbidden. This day, they learned that God provided the fruit for them to eat. It was good and healthy for their bodies.

The sun hid behind the horizon. Stumbling into our rooms, I fumbled in the dark for my lantern. Lighting it in the dark was a test of endurance, similar to the trek to the village. The room suddenly glowed and we could now see the critters that scurried across the floor. I had just settled down for a short power nap when I was summoned to the clinic to attend a birth.

As a midwife, I had attended several births—but never alone and especially alone in a foreign country. Adrenaline accelerated throughout my body as I wondered, *Am I really up to this?*

I did not have my typical supplies nor the medications needed for a birth. My mind flurried around all the things that could go wrong. I asked one of our team members, Dr. J., to assist me with this delivery and he agreed. However, as I entered the clinical area, I learned that I was the only one who could attend to this woman. Dr. J. was not welcome. Traditionally, it was unacceptable for a man to touch another man's wife. Taking a deep breath, I went in to assess the situation and introduce myself to the laboring woman. Dr. J. stayed just outside the door.

I began my initial assessment. The woman was indeed in active labor and about eight centimeters dilated with a bulging bag of water. Standing near her side was a much older woman. The deep furrows on her face and the toughness of her hands revealed a lifetime of struggle and hard work. This woman, soon to be a grandmother, caressed the laboring woman who was her daughter-in-law. Traditionally, for the Miskito Indians, the mother in-law was to be the first to accept the newborn baby. For the proper blessing, she had to be present at the birth.

I had many questions I tried to ask this soon-to-be mother. "Did she have prenatal care?" "Was this her first baby?" "Was she healthy?"

No response. . .

How silly of me, I thought. *Where would she get prenatal care?* I needed to communicate effectively with this woman, and I needed help with translation.

The primary language of Nicaragua is Spanish; but unfortunately, this woman did not speak Spanish. She spoke the tribal language of the Miskito Indians. I needed the English to Spanish translation, then Spanish to Miskito. As the two translators came into the room, our labor and delivery room seemed as small as an American bathroom. Our small room was now packed with a woman in labor, her mother-in-law, two translators and me.

Labor contractions came closer and closer. Between contractions, many of my questions were answered. This mother indeed had had two prenatal care visits at this clinic by a visiting physician. The closest lab was over 200 miles away, and obtainable only by plane, so she did not have any completed lab work. This was her second baby and most important, there was only one baby. The Miskito to Spanish, and Spanish to English translations required great patience. I hoped this woman trusted me to deliver her.

I prayed, *God, guide me and demonstrate your love through me.*

I tried earnestly to communicate with the woman. She would not look at me, but turned away and stared at the wall. I later learned, she did trust me, and her response of turning away was culturally appropriate.

The room was dark, and my small lantern was more of a fire hazard than helpful light. I was afraid of starting a fire. I decided to place the lantern on the floor, to better aid our visual contact with the soon-arriving baby and reduce the possibility of fire. As I lowered the lantern to the floor, I saw many rats running at my feet. I tried not to be alarmed, but I wanted to jump and scream. Somehow, in that cramped room with nowhere to go, I managed to control myself.

Unfortunately, lowering the lantern made it impossible to see the laboring woman's face. Without light, how could I catch the baby? I had attended many births in the United States with minimal lights; but I could always see the mom.

I decided I was close to my breaking point. We needed light. It was getting darker as I fumbled around the packed room.

"Could we find a light?" I asked.

Someone located a gas run generator, but then the fumes were so great, I wondered if I had asked for the right thing. The smell of diesel fuel filled the room, and we all began to cough—including the laboring woman. Dr. J. took the generator, moved it outside the small clinic, and pointed its light in the direction of the tiny window.

Perfect. I could see the mother, she could see me and we all could capture the silhouette of our two translators. The beam of light seemed welcoming and created an ambience of the life yet to be born. I was reminded that God is the light, the way and the path that we should all follow.

I stayed at the woman's side while she continued through the final transition of her labor. The sky again was full of peaceful brilliance. The moon shone vividly through the window; fresh air billowed in. Minutes went by and the mother pushed out the most beautiful and vigorous baby girl. Full head of black thick hair, dark eyes and weighing four kilograms —she came into this world and took her first breath with grace. What a beautiful moment! The sound of the baby's cries floated outside. The other grandmother burst through the clinic door and so did Dr. J.

The placenta delivered without incident and was as perfect as one could imagine. I reflected on my previously anxious thoughts toward the lack of supplies, inefficient prenatal care and possible adverse outcomes. I felt like such a fool. Everything was perfect.

What really matters, I thought, *is the outcome of the baby. All babies are born.*

The mother held her newborn and began to breastfeed immediately. She needed no translation for this natural process. About two hours later, her husband arrived. He looked at her and the baby. He gently took the baby from her and handed her to her grandmother who swaddled her in gathered cloths. He then reached for his bride, gently lifted her from the exam table and carried her home.

I will never forget that breath-taking picture. The husband, a strong and worthy man carrying his wife in the darkness, yet framed by the light of brilliant stars.

The next day, I went to the home. The mother rested in her wooden bed with her baby at her side. Both grandmothers attended them. The home was much like the village clinic we had set up—very few walls and wooden pillars supporting the planked ceiling. Woven cloths that hung from the ceiling divided separate spaces in that one-roomed home. This simple home was filled with family, love and the gift of life.

God is good, all the time.

This birth changed me. I understood clearly that birth happens, no matter where or what the situation. All babies are born, whether we are there to attend or not. Babies are born into the hands of mothers, grandmothers, and even strangers like me.

Women are powerful human beings equipped to give birth. The woman's body is incredible. It changes, adapts and readjusts itself to give birth. The transformation a woman undergoes during pregnancy and childbirth is not an easy process, but an arduous journey of change, pain and submission. One must give up control and give into the forces of labor. By giving up control, a woman can adapt and work with her body to allow birth to happen.

Women surrender themselves to birth just as Jesus surrendered his body on the cross. A mother submits to the labor in order to give birth. Jesus submitted to the cross so that we could be born again. For the Nicaraguan woman and for Christ, the process was not easy, but it was the ultimate act of love.

As I reflected on birth and God's plan for the world, I recalled the Scripture recorded in John 16:21.

"A woman giving birth to a child has pain because her time has come; but when her baby is born, she forgets the anguish because of her joy that a child is born into the world."

Women are incredible.

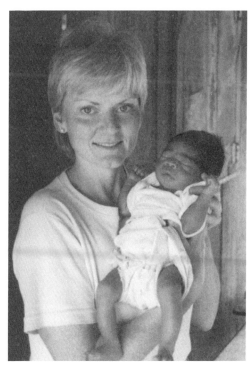

Cathy pictured here with the baby the following day during a home visit.

New Year Baby

Not long after 11:00 p.m., as the party was gaining momentum, my telephone rang. I struggled to hear the caller. The music was so loud.

"Accouchment," the caller yelled. "Acouchement c'est tres difficle, Pouvez-vous venir maintenant?" The national language in Mauritania is French; however, the common language is Arabic. Understanding French with an African-Arabic twist is quite difficult for a Midwestern girl like me. A man was calling for a local midwife who did not speak French, asking me to come to the clinic to aid in a difficult delivery. A first time mother was having difficulty pushing her baby out. The midwives needed help. I responded quickly. Yes, I would come.

When I mention the country, Mauritania, most Americans reply, "Mauri what and where are you talking about?"

The country is a hidden paradise, unknown and uncared about by most Americans. Located on the West coast of Africa, slightly south of Morocco, bordering the Atlantic Ocean on the West and Mali in the East, it resides within the great Sahara desert. I dearly love this country. Despite the difficulty and challenges, I am addicted to the people. I continue to go back for more.

Mauritanian life challenges most Americans. Not just the multi-dialects and religion that stretch us the most, it is the culture and lifestyle that elicits the biggest challenge. In this country, time never progresses. Mauritanians work less, live simply and accept blessings or tragedies as God's will: *Enshallah*. Multi-family homes are the majority, most without running water or electricity. Food and water supplies are scarce due to the desert conditions. Malnutrition and dehydration are an ongoing problem. Hand-dug wells are located throughout the city for people to obtain their daily water supply. Most have their water delivered to their homes by donkeys, pulling fifty-gallon barrels on a cart. This labor-intensive quest for daily water decreases the desire for most Mauritanians to consume or use much water at all.

Mealtime with Mauritanians seems biblical, comparable to the last supper Christ had with his disciples. Partakers sit and recline on a carpet, strategically leaning on their left side, their bodies supported by hand-painted leather pillows, their draping linens concealing their legs centered around a piece of cloth, which transforms into the dinner table. A maiden of the home carries a bowl of water. She bows to participants as each one then cleanses their hands in preparation of the coming meal.

Placed in the middle of the circle of cloth is the piping hot meal of couscous and goat slowly cooling. Using fresh French baguettes, Mauritanians sop up the meat and gravy using only their right hands. The remaining couscous, scoop and cupped in the palm of one's hand, is molded into a ball and eaten until gone. Foreigners like us find eating with our hands part of the adventure. Mauritanians find it hilarious. Thick dripping gravy adheres the couscous between your fingers and the palm of your hand. Ones hand is coated in food, and there are no napkins to wipe it off. Therefore, you lick it off.

Mauritanians just laugh and encourage you to "Mange, mange beaucoup" eat more, eat more. Acculturation for Americans in Mauritanian culture does not come easily. Most ask the same question repeatedly, "Does anyone have a fork or spoon?"

This year, our team arrived in late December and was invited to attend a Fez, a party on December 31st. We excitedly accepted the invitation. New Year's Eve in West Africa, is a celebration of hope and anticipation of what God is giving for the New Year to come. Men religiously attend the Mosque to pray one last time for fortune and fame in the New Year. Our team, the "special guests" at a traditional party, peered through draping fabric of the salon. The festive dancers adorned in bright colors and long veils, swaying to the Arabic music, mystifying us. Heavy aromas of incense and spice penetrated the air as hot bodies danced with the African drums.

My cell phone ringing penetrated the New Year's Eve festivities with an obnoxious ring. I was requested to come to the clinic for a birth. I know I needed to go, and go now. I quickly begged forgiveness from our hosts and began the departure to the clinic. Two of our team members wanted to come along. Walking at night on an unlit road was common here, I hurried to the road to catch a taxi. My phone rang again.

"Accouchement. Accouchment s'il vous plaît se dépêcher." The caller again requested that I come quickly to the clinic. Before I could respond, the phone went dead. Stumbling across rocks, through deep sand, we practically ran full speed to the road.

"Cover your heads, ladies," I shouted as we crossed the dark highway. Culturally, women are not out at night, alone, and especially flagging a taxi. The clock was ticking. Midnight approached. Three American women in an Islamic country desperately tried to find a ride to the clinic. It was not the best of situations.

A curious taxi driver stopped. He was a soft-spoken man who happily gave us a ride to the clinic, especially after hearing our story about an impending delivery. Honking cars clogged the road. The taxi driver did his best to weave through the broken system of vehicles and donkey carts, driving on the side of the road, dodging holes, trash, and avoiding the myriads of people. Despite his efforts, it seemed like an eternity until we arrived at the clinic.

No lights showed the path to the maternity center. Only the moon and stars illuminated the night sky. We again stumbled through dirt-ridden sand and gravel, avoiding the medical waste thrown out for dogs.

As we entered the maternity area, several women greeted us. Tonight was not a good time for long greetings. I stopped to greet them briefly as my mind was racing with the urgency. I continued to move toward the delivery area.

Entering the delivery area, I saw a petite young African woman who was working effortlessly to push her baby out of her body. She was just fourteen. Comforted by two other women, she made no sound. She lay flat on her back, and her veil covered her face as she attempted to push the baby through the birth canal. Springing into action, our small team of women came to her side. Encouraged, she lifted up from the small metal bed, to a semi-sitting position. A small portion of the baby's head began to emerge as everyone shouted words of encouragement in Arabic and French.

The clinic had no trained birth attendant available, only the accouches, women who learn basic delivery skills through an apprenticeship program. They are not nurses, but are instructed in the basic concepts of prenatal care and birth by a seasoned "sage femme" (meaning "wise woman") or midwife. They rarely work alone.

The mother weak, malnourished and very young, continued her attempts to push, but the fetal head was not advancing. As I looked at her eyes, I noted the paleness of her conjunctiva. She was also severely anemic. This was her first baby.

The baby was not advancing into the birth canal. I searched my bag for a vacuum extractor, but it was gone. We needed to start an IV, give her fluids, antibiotics and maybe some Pitocin to aid in stronger contractions. My heart sank, as I pondered how best to aid this poor woman.

Before I could put my bag down; one of the accouches began to push on top of the mother's abdomen with rhythmic movements to move the fetal body through the birth canal. I listened for fetal heart tones with my Doppler. The only thing I could hear were the rhythmic movements of the accouches pushing up and down on the mother's abdomen wall. I could not hear fetal heart tones. Amazingly, with the aid of these barbaric thrusts, the head began to emerge in the birth canal. Donning my gloves, as the head crowned, I delivered the baby. The shoulders slid out as I removed the lifeless baby from the womb.

While drying the baby, using towels to stimulate him, I prayed for his life. "Please God, hear my prayers. Help me."

The room fell silent. There was no pulse. Instinctively, I asked for the time. Someone said, "Just past midnight." I started CPR.

I lifted the baby's lifeless body to a flat service where I could continue to work on him. It was now New Year's Day. "Not today Lord, don't let this baby die, not on the first day of the New Year. Lord, help me, guide, me, send your angels."

The limp baby had no pulse and no respiration. Gently, I held the small baby's chest and back while my thumbs made swift and concise compressions. One-two-three to fifteen then, I bent over the small frame and wrapped my lips around his nose and mouth. I breathed two breaths into the blue baby and watched his chest rise and fall. His body was still limp and cold. I felt lost and could feel every eye in the room watching me.

"Someone please check the mother," I shouted in French, knowing her placenta would soon be delivered.

The baby coughed, took a breath, then stopped breathing. Again, one-two- three …compressions and two breaths. We had a faint pulse. Praise be to God. *Enshallah.* One-minute passed. His apgar score was one; he had a faint pulse of sixty.

Apgar scoring was developed for the sole purpose of identifying the need for resuscitation of a newborn. The scoring is completed at one-minute after birth, five minutes and ten minutes. The highest score achieved is a ten, the lowest is a zero. When babies are not nine or ten at one-minute then action must be taken to aid the baby in full recovery from birth. Again, I resumed CPR.

For a brief moment, I wished I was in America with a trained staff, equipment and life-saving techniques. Radiant heat, oxygen, medications, ventilation and suction could make a different for this first-born son.

Massaging his head, back and chest, I tried to stimulate the baby. Where was that vigorous cry? He was breathing and had a great heart rate but was not moving. His body extended, motionless. I wondered about his brain activity. Had I resuscitated a brain-dead baby? Would be have quality of life? Would he ever play?

The accouches reached for the baby, held him by his feet upside down and slapped his back. The baby still appeared lifeless, despite the improved pulse and steady respirations.

Why wasn't he responding? Could he be cold? Mauritania is a country within the Sahara desert. The temperatures range from warm to hot to hotter. However, this night the temperature was much lower. It felt like winter. It was around fifty degrees fahrenheit, which was very cold to the Mauritanians. Could the baby be cold, I pondered. Unfortunately, there were no thermometers to check his temperature.

The only source of heat was the light bulbs, but skin-to-skin contact was another heat source. I placed the baby on the mother's abdomen, but he continued to lie motionless. He stared at me with blank, black eyes.

"Oh baby, please do not die tonight."

I noticed the sterilizer perched on the cabinet, so I reached across the mother and turned it on. Hurray for electricity. Within moments, the hum of the warming sterilizer coupled with the smell of warming steel filled the room. The warm air radiated across my hands. Reaching over the new mother, I grabbed the blanket and laid it in the sterilizer. Then I reached for the baby and gently laid him on the blanket.

The Mauritanians shouted and yelled at me. I suppose they all thought I was going to sterilize the baby.

I lifted my hand and said in a soft Arabic tone, "Hami-sway, hami-sway" which means, "Please, be patient." We all watched the baby. Tenderly, I stroked his frail body. My hands warmed. The baby grasped my fingers and flexed his arms and legs. He began to cry, like a newborn.

We shouted for joy and praised God. The mother smiled and her mother-in-law stretched to see her newborn son as she recited prayers to Allah. Others bowed immediately in prayer and thanksgiving. The accouches talked in amazement at the changes of the newborn and the importance of heat. Warmed and wrapped snugly in the blanket, our precious New Year's baby was handed to his grandmother for a special blessing.

"Enshallah," they repeated and *"Humdidiallah"* which is "Praise be it God" as they bowed in prayer for the gift of life this New Year's Day.

I know now the strong.

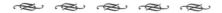

"If any of you lacks wisdom, let him ask of God, who gives to all liberally and without reproach, and it will be given to him." James 1:5

According to the World Health Organization, there are 1.2 physicians, and 6.7 midwives per 10,000 people in Mauritania. The massive shortage of quality health care providers is hampered by the underdeveloped infrastructure of the country. Sadly, it is reported that 10 percent of babies born die at birth, and one in five die within the first five years of life.

Adding to the workforce of health care providers is something we cannot do as easily as we would like to as foreigners. We are faced with multiple barriers such as language, and culture alone. However, educating the current health care providers with basic life skills such as Cardiopulmonary resuscitation (CPR) and Neonatal resuscitation (NRP) can make a huge difference in the statistics of the country. We can teach other providers the basics of NRP so that babies who are not born vigorous have a chance at life. We have an extreme gift of health care knowledge that we can use to teach others in countries like Mauritania. This impact on the health care system can change lives, and demonstrate that each life is worth saving.

Currently, teams have collaborated with Professor Sidi Isslemou OB/Gyn, a national Mauritania physician in country, to train midwives, nurses and physicians. American teams have traveled to Mauritania to train not only NRP but also other skills such as IV's, infection control, CPR, microscopic use and much more. Unfortunately, the training effort has delayed due to the Al Qaeda influence in the area, but we are hopeful it will resume soon. The ministry of health and local police welcome the return of the American health care teams. I am ready.

World Health Organization Fact Sheet:
Newborns—reducing mortality

- Every year nearly 40 percent of all under-five child deaths are among newborn infants, babies in their first twenty-eight days of life or the neonatal period.

- Three quarters of all newborn deaths occur in the first week of life.

- In developing countries nearly half of all mothers and newborns do not receive skilled care during and immediately after birth.

- Up to two-thirds of newborn deaths can be prevented if known, effective health measures are provided at birth and during the first week of life.

The vast majority of newborn deaths take place in developing countries where access to health care is low. Most of these newborns die at home, without skilled care that could greatly increase their chances for survival.

Skilled health care during pregnancy, childbirth and in the postnatal (immediately following birth) period prevents complications for mother and newborn, and allows for early detection and management of problems. In addition, WHO and UNICEF now recommend home visits by a skilled health worker during a baby's first week of life to improve newborn survival. Newborns in special circumstances, such as low-birth-weight babies, babies born to HIV-positive mothers, or sick babies, require additional care and should be referred to a hospital.

Up to two-thirds of newborn deaths could be prevented if skilled health workers perform effective health measures at birth and during the first week of life.

Home visits by a skilled health worker immediately after birth is a health strategy that can increase newborn survival rates. The strategy has shown positive results in high mortality settings by reducing newborn deaths and improving key newborn care practices. While home births are very common in developing countries, only 13 percent of women in these countries receive postnatal care in the first twenty-four hours. Many mothers who give birth in health facilities cannot return for postnatal care because of financial, social or other barriers. The first days of life are the most critical for newborn survival.

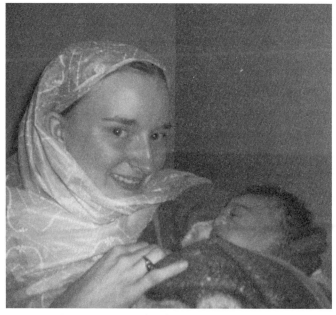

My niece Megan, holding the New Year Baby.

Will You Name Your Baby?

I stared at the fifty-two bug bites on my legs, as my thoughts were endlessly lost in self-pity. I had trekked in North Malawi for several days, providing health care to many needy communities while being eaten alive by massive mosquitoes, flies and other unknown bugs. The red swells on my legs itched like poison ivy. I dared not scratch, because my open wounds would be an easy target for a flaming infection. "I could really use some Benadryl," I thought as I fought the urge to scratch.

My self-absorbed focus ended as I entered the mission clinic to attend to a mother in labor. A tall, lean black woman gently stood in the room, swaying her hips to the rhythm of her contractions. This was not her first baby. She gently moved her body with each contraction, her eyes seemingly void of the birth itself. Beautiful and strong, she would not give in to the mighty forces.

The maternity clinic was a single building in a medical compound. The compound itself spread over about five acres. Each building in the compound had a specific purpose. There was a building for the lab, pharmacy and a different building for consultations etc. All buildings built from cement blocks covered in white paint. Various plants and flowers grew between buildings.

This was not my first trip to Malawi. I had come several times with volunteer health care teams. Our mission was to provide health care to the people and graciously learn the culture. I had come to accept the daily meals of beans and cassava paste. I learned the importance of greeting people as you passed them on a trail, especially the elders. I had also learned that this tropical climate provided a plethora of disease that most health care providers never encountered. Unfortunately, I also had come to understand the importance of taking Malaria prophylaxis to avoid contracting the deadly disease.

The young mother moaned as she labored. Now ready to give birth, she began to push. Putting on gloves, I reached to aid her. The healthcare system lacks having adequate supplies in most developing countries. For example, gloves that the birth attendants use do not fit. They are one-size fits all and very large. I wear size six, which is considered small and their gloves must be at least large enough for size eight or greater. Each glove is similar to a baseball player's mitt. There is a place for a thumb and the second and third finger slide together in the same single slot. The other fingers tucked back because there is no finger areas made for them. The gloves are made of basic plastic, like a sandwich bag. Using these gloves, makes delivering a baby cumbersome for the most obvious reason is that they are two large. After examining a woman you have to hold on to the gloves when completing the exam or they might remain just where you were. Most important, the birth attendant looses the ability to grasp the baby with her fingers tucked back. I prefer to bring my own gloves.

Slowly the dark curly head emerged. His small slender body slid gracefully out of his mother's body. Vigorously he responded to life outside the womb, crying, stretching and breathing air for the first time. His umbilical cord was quickly clamped and cut. His nine-month lifeline could now be a death threat to him, because his mother had just learned she was infected with the HIV virus. No antiviral treatment was provided for her or the unborn baby during her birth simply because it was not available in this part of the world.

His birth was perfect, and he easily transitioned to life. At six pounds, he looked incredible. I looked at the new mother and, reassuringly I said, "God blessed you today with a strong son."

The birth assistant swaddled the newborn in a blanket and handed him to his mother. She did not smile or reach for him, but turned away from him.

I reached for the baby, "It's okay, Mama, I will hold him for you."

I pulled up a stool and sat next to her, so she could see her baby. "So, Mama," I asked quietly in her ear, "what will you name your baby?"

Her vacant dark eyes locked with mine. She paused for a moment, then quietly said in her deep British-African accent, "I will not name him."

I was not sure I had heard her correctly. Maybe she misunderstood my question. The room was busy with staff moving about for a variety of reasons. It was noisy. Maybe I did not understand her response. I was the foreigner and could easily come to the wrong impression, not fully understanding cultural mores. Between her heavy accent and my "American" accent, we could have easier miss-communicated.

I asked again, "Mama, what will you name your baby?"

Again, she quietly replied, "I will not name him."

Confused, I tucked the rooting newborn next to her, and whispered, "It will be okay," while patting her narrow broad shoulders.

Perplexed, I sought out some of the Malawi nurses to find out why she did not want to name her baby. Maybe they planned a baby ceremony later or something, but her demeanor made me think it had to be something else.

"Is it common in Malawi for women not to name their babies?" I asked one of the nurses. Pausing briefly, the nurse looked at me, then turned back to resume her task of cleaning instruments.

Baffled, I wondered, what I was missing, I must have misunderstood something. Maybe the mom was depressed, I really did not know her entire life story. Maybe just the men named the baby. I knew this was commonly practiced in other cultures, but she had no husband.

"Hey ladies," I asked the nurses again but much softer, "why won't she name her baby?"

The birth assistant looked at me, and then tearfully told me the mother's story. "Miss Rose chooses not to give her baby a name, because she fears his death if she names him now, and he dies, his name will not live on. He is supposed to have the name of his father.

"In Malawi your family name is highly valued. The name each child is given determines if he is an heir, a chief or an owner of land. The name one is given is so distinct it truly carves the future for the remaining family. It is important to have a good name in Malawi" she added. After a long pause, she continued, "He must live to carry on the family name of his father. There are no other children."

I asked, "What do you mean, 'if he lives'?" I felt my throat welling in sadness for the life of this mother. I knew she was HIV positive, and I had hope great for her young son . I could only hope that he would somehow, by the grace of God, remain free of the deadly disease of HIV/AIDS.

The assistant shared with me that Rose had been married three times. Her first husband died about five years ago "of sadness" according to the assistant, "because his twin sons and infant daughter died before their first birthday."

"His sadness made him very sick" she shared, "he came to the clinic several times, but the medical assistant assigned to their community could not help him."

After his funeral, Rose had nowhere to go. Her small mud brick home was demolished during the rainy season. The torrential rains destroyed the bricks, turning them to a mud waste similar to waves crashing on a sandy beach. Rose had little income without her husband; therefore, she could not repair the home or purchase food. She worked in the fields of other framers for food. However, her sadness also was great, she missed her husband and children, she also became sick.

Customarily in Malawi, when a man dies, it is the expectation and responsibility of the other men in the family to care for the surviving wife and children. Rose went to live with her husband's oldest brother and he took her in as a wife. Rose gave him a son within the first year. Unfortunately, the baby died at birth and soon after her second husband also died.

"He was sick like his brother," she added, "Rose believed it was 'God's will' that the son died, because his father was not here to care for him."

The assistant finished cleaning the instruments, and began to make tea. Handing me a glass of warm tea, she pulled up another stool and sat down beside me. "Once again, Miss Rose was without a husband or home, so she went to the other brother's home." My eyes welled with tears as I thought about how broken Rose must be, to live a life of such sorrow. I wondered if I could ever be as strong and endure such hardships.

Over the next hour I learned how difficult Rose's life was. The last brother already had two other wives so he was not sure he wanted Rose in his home. He believed she might have brought a curse to their family. The other wives despised her. They demanded she not be allowed to enter their family; however, out of loyalty to his family and Malawi custom, he took her in. He gave her a place to live outside with the chickens, and made her his third wife.

"She was pregnant two more times, but the pregnancies ended in demise. Each time she was pregnant or miscarrying, she came to the clinic for vitamins. The country began to offer free HIV testing to anyone who would agree to the free test. Because Miss Rose had so many babies die, the clinic staff encouraged her to be tested for the HIV infection." she added. Rose agreed and learned that her test was positive. Unfortunately, Malawians do not fully understand the disease; they are quick to fear death. When Rose told her family she had tested positive for HIV, fear and damnation broke loose like a wild horse escaping from his pen.

Rose was immediately outcast from the family. She had nowhere to go as her only family asked her to leave. They believed their fear of the curse had come true. They blamed her for the death of her other husbands and children. They believed she was cursed; therefore, she must die. However, she was now pregnant.

For a short while, Rose lived in the woods until one of the clinic staff invited her to sleep near the clinic. The staff asked the director to have mercy on her and allow her to find an area to stay within walls of the medical compound so that wild animals would not attack her. They knew she was not cursed; rather she was a victim on the HIV virus. The medical staff believed that Rose's family probably all had the virus, but they could only test them and educate them on the disease. The family refused testing; only Rose was tested. The clinic director had compassion for Rose and designated an area where she could camp behind the buildings.

In exchange for her simple refuge, Rose daily gathered trash, burned it and kept the clinic floors clean. The staff shared their food with her from the small portions they brought for themselves.

I sat motionless. I could not speak. I couldn't even think. I was stunned. I turned my head to glance back at Rose. She was breastfeeding her baby.

Although I understood only slightly, the brokenness of Rose's life, I also knew the importance of this young baby's name. He was alive, and God had a great purpose for his life. I believed the words of Jeremiah,

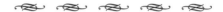

"Before I formed you in the womb I knew you, before you were born I set you apart; I appointed you as a prophet to the nations." Jeremiah 1:5

Malawi is located in southern Africa and is among the African countries hardest hit by HIV. Approximately 930,000 people live with HIV in Malawi, 52 percent of whom are women fifteen years of age or older. In 2007, there were approximately 68,000 deaths due to AIDS among adults and children in Malawi, and approximately 560,000 AIDS orphans. HIV especially impacts women and children. At the end of 2007, there were approximately 91,000 Malawian children living with HIV and 73,000 HIV-positive pregnant women, of whom only 32 percent received some form of antiretroviral prophylaxis. **(HIV/AIDS statistics from UNAIDS.)**

HIV has become the largest killing disease in the history of the world. More people have died from AIDS than all wars combined. It is a secret killer looming in Africa, China and other countries while remaining out of sight and mind in the developing countries.

The problem is real. It is also growing. Next to abstinence, education is the number one prevention. Unfortunately, the cultural climate of any given country is difficult to change; Malawi is losing a generation. Life expectancy is not long enough in Malawi for grandparents to take in the surviving orphans. These children are going to mission orphanages.

We can make a difference in countries like Malawi by ongoing education, and free testing of HIV to the Malawian people. We can also tell the story of many women like Rose who succumb to AIDS and never really understand why. Their voices, the innocent victims of HIV/AIDS, must be heard across the globe for changes to occur. Rose's life had value, her life is being echoed today, change is happening and treatment for HIV infected mothers is beginning to penetrate Malawi.

On my next visit to Malawi, I learned that Rose had died. Her son was living with Christian missionaries in an orphanage. To their knowledge, the young boy has remained HIV negative. I never learned his name.

"A good name is more desirable than great riches; to be esteemed is better than silver or gold." Proverbs 22:1

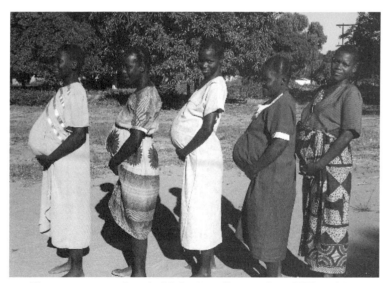

Five pregnant mothers in Malawi, sadly two of are HIV positive.

River Of Life

Stepping out of my cabin the intense humidity and heat overwhelmed me. Waves from the river gently tossed the riverboat from side to side while the growl of the engine irritated my pounding head. The air was thick and murky and fumes of exhaust lingered like the smoke stench from a fat old cigar. Temperatures soared at least ninety degrees with 100 percent humidity producing beads of sweat on my brow. The sun peered over from the horizon mysteriously blinding views of the massive river surrounding us. This was the mighty Amazon River. I was not sure if I should be afraid or excited, so I retreated to my cabin in search of Tylenol.

Flying into Peru the night before, our health care team anxiously boarded the riverboat as it quickly departed for our first destination, a community of Amazonian people. Our team was composed of a variety of health care professions as part of a Mercy & Truth Medical Missions outreach. We had met briefly prior to leaving the USA, now we were traveling together into the uttermost parts of the world.

The night sky and massive starts illuminated my feet like a lantern. Locating my cabin, I instinctively dropped my luggage where I stood and dove onto the bed. It did not take long for the boat to rock me to sleep as a newborn baby nestled next to his mother. I was exhausted. Major fatigue swept over me, having traveled all day to arrive at this remote destination in Iquitos, Peru. I slept.

Morning came quickly. The abrupt change in climate coupled with long travel ignited a migraine in my head. My stomach churned with nausea, with each pounding sensation in my brain. I hate headaches. The breakfast bell ran, summoning our team to the dining room. I found my Tylenol, swallowed down a couple of tablets and made way to the lower level. Breakfast did not sound so good. Being the team leader, I knew I needed to greet our team despite how good I felt. Entering the room the array of fresh fruits and fish filled the air. The room had a beautiful buffet of foods lining a small corner of the ship. The bright colors and variety of unknown delectable's lured me to taste anyway. Incredible flavors danced on my palate, fresh mango, papayas, sweat banana and many herbs captivated me to indulge. I had never tasted such succulent ripe fruit. The rich taste of these new flavors overwhelmed the sensations in my mouth. I was in heaven. I briefly thought about the produce back at home on our grocery shelves. It was not the same. The taste here was incredible.

The boat soon docked near a sandy beach. Our curious American eyes looked out at the village around us. Trees and brush densely populated the area except for occasional dwellings and pathways. Wooden piers mounted in the miry river edges held high the homes of many Amazonian families. The homes were similar to small cabins snuggled amidst a tree line. Held together by hand carved tongue in groove boards, the homes had two-three rooms apiece. The rooms designed for sleeping, eating and cooking had open air windows covered in woven brush. A ladder from the ground gave entry to each home onto a small platform or porch. Small livestock such as chickens, monkeys and rabbits strategically hoisted in woven cages hung from the roof over the platform. Larger livestock, mainly pigs or goats, were fenced beneath the home, between the piers. The Amazonian people peered back at us with their large brown eyes from behind their canvas windows.

The SHOFAR sounded. The low long tones of the ancient Hebrew trumpet were used to announce the arrival of the health care team to the village. The missionaries would stand at the highest point on the riverboat and sound the SHOFAR. The echoing tones would travel with the river as far as one could see. It produced silence around us as it sounded over the treetops. Soon, people appeared from their homes, out of the dense jungle at the call knowing the doctors and nurses had arrived. Dugout canoes silently slid through the water to our boat to dock and enter. Within minutes, we were surrounded by hundreds of families waiting to be seen for a variety of illnesses and maladies.

Quickly, the riverboat transformed into a clinic. The dining room became a surgical suite covering the tables with sterile drapes. Lower levels of the boat became a pharmacy and the additional cabins became exam rooms. Triage initiated by the nurses on land with the boat's wooden plank admitting those whom had registered. Hundreds of Amazonians appeared and waited. One by one, they received needed health care for parasites, malaria, and illnesses not cured by rain forest herbs.

Clinic hours initiated at daylight and most often closed as the sun set beyond the horizon. At the end of the day, while enjoying fresh Amazonian fish, our team debriefed. We discussed the many ailments and tropical diseases that were presented with our Amazonian clients. We discussed and learned about the variety of local treatments people used for relief of their symptoms. Our first day finished after seeing over 500 families. My headache was gone. I had learned so much today.

Early the next morning, I asked for the local health care providers, midwives or healers to join us for consultations. During our outreaches, I often call on the "local health care providers" and midwives to come and meet with me and any other women of the community. We could learn so much from them. All of the American health care team desired to learn some of the secrets of the Amazon herbs and treatments. The mayor of the village asked for the "shaman" or witch doctor to come. He refused. However, the two village midwives came, and they expressed a desire to learn from us. I hoped they could teach me.

The midwives shyly presented papers to me to review. The documents neatly folded between cardboard sleeves contained a certification that they had attended and completed training to be "official" birth attendants. They received their training from a government hospital about 100 miles from their village. The women proudly showed these documents to our team. Neither of them could read or write their own Peruvian dialect or Spanish, but had both received training in birth. We were all very proud of them and openly welcomed them to join our healthcare team. Immediately, we began to share birth stories including birth positions and treatments with each other. It did not take long for us to be friends and laugh at each other despite our vast difference in rendering services.

We quickly learned that the Amazonian midwives are talented and creative women who use many different plants and herbal remedies to conquer just about every imaginable ailment. They were the village health care providers. Learning from their predecessors about healings and births, they maintained the tradition of their ancestors and were expected to keep the traditions alive by teaching apprentice midwives. Training without textbooks or lessons, the inexperienced engage in a symbiotic relationship with their mentors absorbing details of their work, side by side. This designation of being a midwife in the community is a role of vast importance.

The midwives shared that they rarely received any form of money for their work. Payment for services rendered varied based on the value of the family. Sometimes they were invited to a celebratory meal at the home of the family, and given livestock such as chicken or a monkey. One midwife shared she was given a western treat, a Coca Cola for delivering a baby. Midwives attended births day and night even for struggling animals. They shared stories about aiding a difficult breech or twin deliveries of local goats, pigs and cattle. The Amazonian midwives' hands are valued as birth protectors in this community.

The midwives also shared that they collect and grow plants for infusions and teas to facilitate labor and birth. They have a plant for birth, bleeding, healing, breast milk and on and on. During labor, they give the mother tea to drink for strength. If her labor slows, they speed it up with other teas. Walking through their gardens, I wanted so badly to understand more about each plant they grew, so I took many pictures. They seemed so knowledgeable despite the fact none of them could read or write their own spoken language.

It was not long after we met that one of the midwives was summoned to attend a woman in labor. Hurriedly she gathered a sachet of herbs while explaining that women in the Amazon will often continue their daily work until the pain is too unbearable as they labor. Then call for the midwives. Therefore, she must move quickly or she may miss the birth. She invited me to attend. I jumped at the opportunity.

Responding to a home delivery in the Amazon seemed exciting and scary. There are no hospitals or clinics available, all of the women delivered their babies at home. There were no other options. We trekked through the thick jungle passing a few homes along the way. There was no obvious trail or path to follow. The midwife knew the way. I was hopeful our destination was not far because the long trek through the jungle left me confused as to my whereabouts. My eyes constantly watched for snakes dangling from the trees, or sloths reaching for my head. I wished I had some sort of markers or Reese's pieces to leave behind so I could find my way back. I laughed at my own nervousness knowing the Reese's pieces worked in the movie E.T. as they lured an alien. I definitely felt like that alien in a foreign land now, lost in the jungle. Surely, they would walk me back to the boat, I hoped.

Approaching a home deep within the thicket, we arrived at our destination. The house was wooden, standing on stilts with two very large pigs fenced immediately below. We climbed the rugged hand carved ladder about fifty feet high to the platform home. It had a small sturdy porch leading to a large open room covered by a thatched roof. The walls only about three feet high easily accepted the warm river breeze. The smell of fresh rains and flowers filled the room. The sounds of birds, bugs, and chickens saturated the background. Draped on the walls were woven reed mats. There were no beds, just a single mat lying across the plank floor. The mat was beautiful. Blended colors of fuchsia pink and teal green reeds decorated it. It was made specifically to welcome the new baby. Standing near was a woman, clearly in labor.

The young mother was beautiful. Her long black hair draped over her tiny body as she slowed moved her hips from side to side. Her low moans were music to our ears, the music that led the dance of labor and love. Mixing tea on a small pit stove, the midwife handed it to the mother. She sipped the freshly made tea of herbs and continued in her dance. The midwife chanted, and sang as the mother moaned and danced. The sound of rain penetrated the air as she swayed her body with the waves of contractions.

Encouraging the mother to drink more tea, the midwife's hands began to massage the mother. Using a tin of lard as lotion, the midwife applied it in a circular motion to the abdomen and back of the dancing women. She moved with the mother to not break the rhythm of her labor. She explained to me that fresh lard is used as an emollient for women in labor and is believed to help the baby "slide out" easily. While the midwife massaged, the mother drank her tea and continued her dance. I sat quietly observing and wondering what would happen next. Her body shifted and swayed to comfortable positions with each contraction.

The mother moaned in song and danced. For most women, as their labor progresses and their babies descend into the birth canal, they assume a position that is most comfortable to them and begin to push their babies out. Instinctively this mother knelt to the floor. The midwife helped her steady herself. She never touched the woman's vagina, perineum, or "checked her" cervical dilation. Explaining to me it is taboo to touch women in the genital area in this Amazonian culture. They believe that a curse could be cast upon them or the baby if they touched her. The midwife shared that they rarely perform a vaginal exam to determine a woman's progress with labor. They would only assess her if she had a concern.

As the mother squatted, the baby emerged from her body. She then gracefully, as if she had done this several times, lowered her body to the freshly woven mat and on to her side. The new mother reached and lifted her newborn to her chest as he took in his first breath. Immediately the midwife secured and tied the umbilical cord and swiftly severed the cord with the family's knife. A few minutes passed and the midwife then helped the mother back into a squatting position, and the placenta delivered onto the same mat.

Within minutes, the birth mat began to fill with blood. The blood ran to the edges, soaking the reeds along the way. It was more than a trickle of blood, it seemed like a river, a river of life flowing from her. The midwife encouraged the mother to lie down and breastfeed the baby. Breastfeeding helps the body release Oxytocin. The natural release of Oxytocin from the woman's body from a nursing baby would aid in reducing the blood flow. My heart started to race as I watched this mother bleed. I could feel my own adrenaline surge in concern for this mother. I wanted to do something.

Instinctively, I reached out and began to massage the mother's uterus. Blood clots emerged but the bleeding did not stop. While supporting the uterus, I massaged the upper portion in hopes it would clamp down and stop bleeding. The bleeding continued. Doing my best at sign language, I asked the mother if I could look at her bottom and see where the bleeding was coming from. She agreed. I grabbed some towels, and used them as gauze to absorb the blood so I could look for an area of bleeding. Using my headlamp for light, I searched for the source of bleeding. The bleeding slowed with the compression of the towels just long enough for me to see the cause. She had endured a severe laceration as she gave birth. The laceration extended deep within her. This is why she was bleeding so much. She needed suturing.

I motioned to the midwife for her to look at the area. She glanced briefly and went back to the baby. Her objective was to get that baby to breastfeed. Again, I motioned to the midwife and using my hands, I pointed to the new mother's laceration. I also acted like I was sewing trying to get her to see this woman needed to be sutured. The midwife looked at the laceration and intuitively reached for her sachet. I was hoping she was going to pull out some sutures.

Sorting through her herbs, she picked out a few of them and set the others aside. Crushing them with a primitive mortal and pedestal, the herbs quickly transformed into a fine dust. Using the same bowl, she added a handful of the lard and mixed it into the finely broken herbs. A smell penetrated the air as if fresh cheese and sauerkraut were fermenting in the room. Removing the packing I had employed with the towels, the midwife placed the poultice as if painting a tapestry and leaving none of the canvas untouched. Then she asked the mother to straighten her legs and keep them together for the next several hours. I watched and waited. The bleeding stopped.

I sat back and watched the new mother gently caress and feed her baby. She seemed clueless to the bleeding she endured and the severity of the situation.

The birth mat's purpose was now complete. The mother moved to a clean mat with her newborn son. The birth mat was firmly rolled and secured closed with twine in preparation of its disposal. The midwife placed the rolled and bound mat aside for the family to dispose of it. The family would burn the mat in twenty-four hours or less as a ritual. This burning signifies a new spirit is lifted in celebration of the new life. Amazingly, the mats are also used for the dying in the same manner. They will wrap their deceased family members in the same type of mat and offer their bodies in a cremation type of ceremony. These people believed that burning of the body lifts the spirit to the heavens.

Prior to leaving this home and venturing back to the boat, my curiosity mounted. I wanted badly to take just one more look at this woman's bottom. Being denied the opportunity, I respected the culture by not pressing my concerns any further, but realizing the consequences that could occur. I was compelled as a woman to be sure to teach others about child birth and hemorrhage. I never learned if her laceration healed or she resumed bleeding. I can only hope.

This experience brings a strong correlation to the midwives of Egypt. In Exodus 1:19 the midwives reported to Pharaoh that some women deliver fast and well as the Hebrews.

"The midwives answered Pharaoh, 'Hebrew women are not like Egyptian women; they are vigorous and give birth before the midwives arrive.'"

Birth can happen very fast. It is highly recommended that women always have a trained birth attendant present. It is not safe for women and their babies to deliver without trained attendants. Sadly, thousands of women die each year as a result of childbirth. The majority of maternal deaths occur in developing countries and regions like the Amazon. There is a strong call for women to give birth with the aid of trained birth attendants. The world health organization has published a fact sheet on skilled birth attendants that can be found at: WHO/MPS/08.11 World Health Organization FACT SHEET.

Even in the Bible there are reported deaths after childbirth by the midwives. Unfortunately, the number one cause of maternal death globally is a result of post partum hemorrhage according to the World Health organization. Women who die from hemorrhage are most likely giving birth alone and without the aid of a skilled childbirth attendant. Most trained birth attendants are able to identify and stop hemorrhage. Unfortunately, many do not have adequate supplies like the midwives of this Amazonian region.

These midwives lacked the supplies needed to close and suture a bleeding laceration. Herbs can be used to stop the bleeding, but they cannot close a laceration. We can learn from these midwives the value of using herbs and they can learn from us how to close wounds.

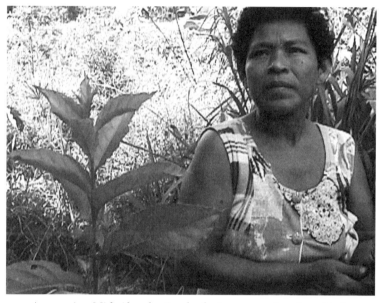

Amazonian Midwife selecting herbs in preparation for a birth.

Teach One

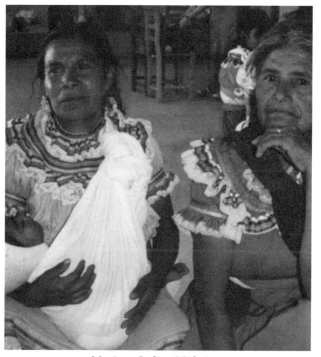

Mexican Indian Midwives.

My very first medical mission outreach was unforgettable and became a major pathway of God's gifting purpose in my life. Our team was the first medical mission team from our church. We left Kansas City by car, and drove to the San Antonio, Texas area to meet up with the rest of the team. Together, we traveled in a small convoy for an additional two days by to a very remote area of Western Mexico. As we came closer to our destination the road conditions worsened. The last five hours of driving were horrific to say the least.

Boulders lined the road between large crevasses, deep holes and tortuous treacherous pathways. These "roads" as they called them guided us high into the mountains. Fatigue, profound nausea and major headache swept over me like a vicious plague coupled with the fear of falling off the mountain. There was nowhere to rest, relieve my nausea or even have access to medications to help. Tightly packed in an old suburban in much need of a muffler and shocks I sat upright like a sardine with fifteen other tired, stinky Americans and Mexicans. I remember the game we played in high school on how many people we could cram into a bus bathroom. This ride seemed almost as challenging.

My frustration mounted as the waves of nausea surfed my body. "What possessed me to pay to go through this" I thought, "I must have been psycho to sign up for this." I know God had a plan for me, to serve His people with the gift of health care that I had received. What I never intended on enduring was the conditions of pain and ridiculousness. I did not know that I would physically suffer like this, and it would be so hard even before we got there. Nor did I ever imagine riding like a tightly packed jar of peaches smothered in hot syrup ready to be canned.

It didn't take long to have the welling grow from my stomach to the back of my throat. It was only a matter of time before I knew I would "blow." The pressure and need to throw-up surmounted to the point of my meek request to "please pull over, I am going to puke." Of course, the driver refused to stop, I was not sure if it was a "man thing or what." I knew I was going to hurl very soon and something had to give. Maybe they thought I was joking around or "just a wimpy girl," maybe I was. I resorted to primitive manners. Grabbing a nearby plastic grocery bag, I hung the handles on my ears, much like a horse eating his oats, leaving my nose out for air. Turning my head to the side of the truck, I lost my lunch several times while we ascended into the depths of this mountain. Frustration, embarrassment and disgust came over me and I again pondered on the idea why I had agreed to go on this outreach, it was not fun. Surly God had a big plan for me, because I wasn't even to the destination, and I was ready to go back home.

It was dark as we drove onto the final plateau, about 14,000 feet high within the Sierra Mountains. Bonfires seen blazing in the distance led us to the final resting place where we would set up camp. Exhausted we all managed to untangle our bodies from the truck and crawl out. We were welcomed by a crowd of about 100 people, clapping and singing next to the fire. They stood together smiling to greet these new strangers in their world. Stares of excitement and fear mounted their faces as we approached them. The raging fire provided a glow of light across the welcome team. Beautiful men and women stood greeting us. Few had shoes. Women were dressed in traditional clothing of peasant-like shirts with an embroidered pattern of vibrant color flowing over full layered, multi-colored skirts. They were stunning. We had never met Tarahumara Indians, indigenous to this area of Mexico, and they had never met Americans.

The welcome ended quickly as we were scavenging the truck for our gear and setting up camp. The only light source we had was the bonfire and the million stars that illuminated the sky. The truck was quickly unpacked, and like a blind man we felt for our backpacks, tents and sleeping bags. Amazingly, my little tent popped up without a hitch. Doing my best to remove rocks and sticks from beneath, I set the tent on solid ground for the night stay. Sleeping bags rolled out and I jumped in, my roommates soon followed. I was sharing a tent with two other women, both of whom were seasoned medical missionaries from Georgia. Their southern drawls seemed to be a comfort to my Midwestern inexperienced twang. We instantly became friends. Within just a few short minutes they both were snoring, and I was drifting into "la la land."

Morning came quickly; we truly had just laid down when the sun began to rise beyond the horizon. Scuffling of feet and laughter of children could be heard. Peeking my head ever so slightly out of my sleeping bag, I noticed a remarkable difference in the air temperature. "Oh my goodness it is cold" I stated while watching my breath billow from my mouth. Reaching for my bag through the open door of the tent I searched for my clock. I fumbled with an unopened bottle of Pepsi, frozen in my bag, as my hand found my clock. It was six-o'clock in the morning. Instinctively, I nestled back into my sleeping bag, pulling it up and over my head while shivering. My roommates both rolled in close to me and gave me there body warmth. The effect was incredible as I drifted back to sleep.

When breakfast was ready, our group walked up a slope to a nearby mud brick adobe home. Winded we trekked this small pathway. We were obviously a group of flat-landers, breathing heavily with each step. A freshly cut log became our resting place to enjoy freshly made corn tortillas, beans and eggs, and catch our breath. I am not sure if it was the incredible scenery that captivated me more or the aroma of brisk mountain air that seemed so fresh and pure. It seemed like a glimpse of heaven here. I sat motionless as I watch the Indian women grind more corn, mix the meal with water and slap them into tortillas. They performed this task with such grace. Eagerly, I jumped up from the log and joined them in their outdoor kitchen, perching on the ground to watch more closely. They welcomed me into their covey.

None of these women spoke Spanish, and neither did I so we were off to rocky start. But, there is something to be said about women in the kitchen, even if the kitchen is basically a fire outside. Now, one would automatically think that we would all chatter like chickens, not exactly, I did not speak their Aztecan dialect and they did not speak English. We talked with our hands and faces. I watched their hands skillfully work the cornmeal, they were masters. I motioned for me to try. Openly they accepted me into their kitchen, their safe zone. They taught me, they laughed at me, and we laughed together. I made odd shaped thick tortillas, and they ate them anyway. On our first day, we became friends without speaking a word.

I was soon summoned to come help set up clinic, so down the slope I went. Our tents were used for the clinic rooms, and pharmacy. Transforming camp was easy. Since this was my very first medical outreach, I was more of a "helper or gopher" than anything else. I was given the task of "do this, do that, go here and go there." I can do that! We were ready to see our patients within an hour, it was nearly 8:00 a.m. by now, and we were ready. We had two tents set up for consultations, one for the pharmacy, and an area behind the truck for the dentist. It was perfect. The announcement was made that the clinic would begin with the tribal chief while we stopped to thank God for these people and our ability to serve them.

One by one we began our consultations. Each person was seen for whatever ailment they presented with. Most had complaints of pain somewhere in their bodies. I understood this more as I observed their day to day life of chopping wood, sleeping on the ground, and carrying water alone. Every person received vitamins and parasite treatments. My role was to help the pharmacist count out the vitamins, Tylenol and many other medications we were giving. I also kept our dentist supplied with lidocaine as he pulled teeth on every single person he saw.

The dentist, a Mexican man who had a desire to impact his own people by aiding in dental care, joined our team as we entered the mountains. The campsite dental operatory was impressive to say the least. Every person he saw sat on a gasoline can and leaned their heads back on a truck while he examined their teeth. No electricity for instruments or lighting, the dentist viewed their mouths by using a head lamp illuminated from the sunlight. He worked endlessly on each person, using primitive hand tools to complete the tasks of tooth extraction and repair. He truly went above and beyond to serve these people. His work impacted my heart. I stood ready to aid him in any capacity I could and was amazed at his servant's heart.

Dr. John Powell, a pediatrician was our medical team leader. He had served on several medical missions outreaches in multiple countries and started an organization called Evangelism task Force is Wayside Georgia specifically for medical teams. He was amazing. This guy acted so natural and "at home" with the idea of using his medical knowledge for people he had never met. He never complained, and always was ready to see "one more" even when the sun dropped below the horizon. His endless service captivated my heart. I saw a living example of Christ's service on earth through Dr. Powell. I wanted to know more.

My devotion that night reflected the attitude of serving God's people with the gifts he has bestowed upon us. I realized on this day that God had set me up for a purpose in healthcare. I too, had been given a gift of health care knowledge in nursing and I needed to use my gift for His people freely as it had been given to me. I reflected on the verse is Matthew 10:8 to heal the sick, for freely I have received and freely I can give. Crawling back into my tent, I asked God, "How can I do this, I am just a nurse, not a doctor or dentist, how can I serve you with the gifts you have given me?"

The following day, my headache started to leave me, finally. This day, I bolted out of my tent to trek the slope and aid our new friends in the kitchen. They had a place ready for me when I arrived. Together we made tortillas. I had yet to master the skill. As I sat on the mountain side looking down at the camp I noticed people everywhere. There must have been 1,000 or so Tarahumara Indians that had come overnight to our site. I soon learned that they had walked all night to come to our clinic today. I wondered then, how could we see them all? There were so many.

Our clinic camp transformed easier today with some new additions. We set up new tarps to aid in relief from the hot sun to the waiting crowd. We also set up a tarp where the local pastor shared the gospel. This area was separated from the clinic and the waiting area so as not to impose the gospel on anyone not desiring it. Many sat in his tent and listened for hours as the clinic saw hundreds of families this day.

That day, I spent time aiding Dr. Powell. I had hoped to gain some health care wisdom from him. Client after client presented him with a variety of ailments, all wanted something for pain. I soon learned most people just needed basic health care, something nurses are good at. They needed teaching on hygiene, infection, and teeth. They needed someone to care. It did become apparent that there was a common thread among women. Many had asked how they could stop being pregnant. They talked about being pregnant a lot, and many babies dying at birth. At first I thought there must be a problem with translation, surely they knew.

At the end of each clinic day we debriefed on unusual presentations, problems, and what remained in our pharmacy. Two major concerns were raised, one being the amount of head lice that was seen among the tribal people and the need for health care education. It was decided that the next day we would set up two additional stations, one for head lice treatments, and one for women. Exhausted, I crawled into my tent realizing my headache was finally gone, and falling into a deep sleep, I still asked God, "How can I be effective? How can I use my gifting for your people? Show me God, I prayed."

I slept hard, not moving at all. I awoke suddenly with a stiff back, needing to stretch, move or something. Reaching for my clock I saw it was four o'clock in the morning and I was wide awake. I closed my eyes and tried to go back to sleep, I couldn't. Therefore, searching for my flash light, and finding it under my sleeping bag, I unzipped the tent and crawled out. Careful not to walk into another camp area, the Tarahumara families were everywhere; I tiptoed to the edge of the plateau and begin to climb the side of the mountain. There was a moon tonight, I could see every step I took, and it was beautiful.

The night air filled my nostrils as I trekked slowly through the rugged terrain. I must have been a bit crazy to be out alone, in the wilderness. I did not feel alone though, I felt driven. I found some boulders, perched up on them and was still before God. I sat still, looking at the vast universe in awe and recited the verse of Psalms 46:10 in my mind, **"Be still, and know that I am God; I will be exalted among the nations, I will be exalted in the earth."** I sat still and prayed to God to be exalted among the nations now, in this village with these people and to bless them. I prayed for the work that was being done, I prayed for guidance and wisdom as I was so drawn into His service but did not know how I could be useful, I sat still and waited on God. The sun began to rise, it was breathtakingly beautiful. I felt the majesty in this place, I knew God was here.

I scurried back to camp and trekked the hill once again to sit with my lady friends. Today I mastered a perfect flat tortilla. Great praise and adoration was given to me as the tortilla was browned on the camp fire. "My tortilla" was then given to me to eat and it indeed was good.

Clinic was delayed today so we could initiate head lice treatments at the river. Men, women and children all came as we dipped their heads in the mountain river, applied lindane, and gave instructions on when to wash. Many came and were happy to stand in the icy water. Announcements were made that a special women's meeting would be occurring soon under the tarp. Women began to gather under the tarp ready to learn.

Meeting women in developing countries is often a challenge due to many barriers keeping them from the developing world. Rarely did we find Tarahumaran women who spoke any Spanish. Language barriers alone kept them from conversing and growing in the nearby cities. Most had never ventured far from their mountaintop homes, only their husbands braved the new world. Geographic barriers hampered any formal education for most women allowing them to obtain any type of formal education or attend school. However, our classroom was full of women who desired to learn more from their foreign counterparts. They came, and waited ready to indulge in knowledge.

Our meager classroom was packed full of women alone. Many men wanted to attend also, but were not dismayed when we requested that only women be present. Our desire in having a "women only" meeting was to decrease any inhibition or embarrassment on asking questions. Not knowing all the taboos of this tribal society, we had hoped not to break any by exposing a lifestyle unacceptable in our health care world. The men understood and openly welcomed their wives, mothers and daughters to attend what the referred to as the "health classroom."

Class started with an introduction of our women's health care team. Our groups consisted of one physician, three nurses (including myself) and two nonmedical women who had excellent experience as mothers. Utilizing two translators, Aztecan to Spanish, Spanish to English, to the health care team and back again, we began discussing basic health care topics. Hand washing, wound care, and nutrition opened the door of discussion. Amazingly our Tarahumara friends were not shy at all but conversed and began asking questions in great detail.

It did not take long for these women to begin to feel confident enough to start asking some very poignant questions. Several women were discussing among themselves and finally stood up and asked three point blank questions, "why to bleed every month, how can we   stop having so many babies and why did so many die in childbirth." Wow, I actually thought we must have a problem with translation, so we asked them again in a different way what were the questions they wanted answered. Again, it was repeated, "why to bleed every month, how can we stop having so many babies and why did so many die in childbirth." Didn't they know or understand why they had menstruation, how they got pregnant and the process of childbirth? Our sessions were now "cut out" for us. The challenge was to effectively teach these women about the normal processes in their bodies despite the barriers of language and culture we were embarking on.

Over the next four hours we discussed the process of growth and development, maturity and aging in both the women and men. Using the land we stood on as a black board I drew pictures in the dirt with a stick. Sure some laughed, but most intently watched and asked more and more questions. The process just to get through "the basics" of reproduction seemed to last longer than expected using the translators, but there was no faster way. Time passed quickly, as the afternoon sun began to beat down on our classroom. Questions arose from our indigenous audience specifically about the actual conception process. The women repeatedly asked "is this how we get pregnant?" We discussed the details of conception, God's plan for a husband and wife to have sex, family planning in great detail more than I will write about now in this chapter. The women began to chatter amongst themselves. They recited to us and themselves how, when and why they were getting pregnant. The women requested a break so they could share this news with their husbands; therefore, we agreed this would be a great time for a break. Following the break we shared with the women we would discuss childbirth.

Commencement of the afternoon session drew a larger crowd. The men now wanted to sit in the classroom with the women. It was obvious that most of the women left the morning session and began telling their husbands everything they had learned. I was thrilled, it was an obvious demonstration that our teaching was effective, or at least we had hoped. I also was glad to see that the women were openly discussing what that had learned. Their excitement and new knowledge spread through the camp like a wild fire. The men wanted to understand more about their bodies and the implications that childbirth was having on their families. They came to "hear that what the women were saying was true." We agreed for the men to attend the afternoon session. Before we could even begin, we had an unexpected visitor.

The curandera, or tribal healer, came and began waving his stick over our tents and chanting. He slowly moved throughout the camp, not missing any area. The Tarahumara people ignored him, but I could not. It was hard not to watch him as he became quite a distraction, at least to me. I wondered what he was doing. The tonality of his voice was harsh and quite loud at times. His large stick would wave and thrash at times pointing at people, our medicines and our supplies. Motioning to Dr. Powell, I asked him in English of course, what this guy was up to, because I was beginning to get scared. We were encouraged to keep on meeting and do our best to ignore him. I silently prayed that God would cover us with protection against evil, against witch craft, and whatever this guy's purpose was. I also asked God to help this healer to find favor in our work and join us in health care.

Our meeting continued into the topic of childbirth. We determined very quickly that families were very private. Within the family unit there was a great concern for the well being of anther individual, they cared about each other. We asked them to tell us about childbirth for women. The men shared that many of their wives had died because of childbirth. Most died after the baby was born, leaving them to care for a newborn alone as well as any other children. They revealed that the women often would live for about a week then become very sick with fever and confusion prior to dying. One man shared that three of his wives had died in childbirth and wondered if God had put a curse on his family. Hearing these stories brought tears to our eyes. We asked them to share in more detail what happens during labor, birth and the immediate postpartum period.

Labor was experienced alone by most women. Sadly we listened to story after story of what women experience in childbirth. It was a private event, no formal birth attendant came. They were hours from any hospital making complications something they had to endure. The women relied only on their own families for assistance, as needed, and when requested.

Women would stay in their homes once labor began until they delivered and were strong enough to leave the home. They did not gather water from the river, cut fire wood, prepare meals or any other tasks during labor. The husband would learn of their labor because they would not perform any tasks. That is if the husband was at the home and not hunting or going to another village. The women did not ask for help, even from other women as it was a sign of weakness and also considered taboo for others to watch a woman give birth.

They believed labor would last one to seven days, depending on the stars and the strength of medicine provided by the curandera. Sometimes the curandera would be summoned to prepare them a drink or special paste from beans to eat that would cause them to sleep.

"Sleep would either make the baby come faster or slow the baby's coming down. When the baby was closing to coming, they would usually squat on their feet and hands to help the baby come out" they shared. "After the baby was born and birth was complete, they would cut the cord by smashing it between rocks. Then they would lie down with the baby on a mat and rest."

The mat, woven specifically by the mother-to be prior to the birth of her baby, was to collect fluids from the birth. It is made from tall green grass that is dried and stored until the birth occurs. After delivery, the mat is rolled up and burned. Women nodded their heads in agreement. Their stories left me speechless for a brief time.

My mind raced with ideas and concerns of how I or anyone on our team could best impact their lives today. Realizing we had major cultural differences I knew that extreme cautiousness must be utilized when discussing lifestyles and possible changes to prevent death. Often, I have seen many people take on the "know it all approach" as if we ruled the earth in knowledge and wisdom. Today, education of conception alone was profoundly life changing in these tribal people. Now we were discussing childbirth in an area where there were no hospitals, no medications, no electricity, no running water and not even a trained birth attendant, the comfort level to most Americans. We were stretched into extreme acculturation.

Being a "rookie," I sat silently as a learner myself, as a Mexican physician and other team members made incredible suggestions to aid these women in childbirth. She understood more of their culture than I had as a newcomer in the area. Initially, the women were encouraged to talk to one another and others women in the community about what they were learning. They were encouraged to take this new knowledge and channel it into wisdom for their community while complementing them on their strong work ethic and family bonds.

The classroom turned to focus on birth and the importance of safety for the mother and the baby. The Tarahumara women listened intently. Basic yet descriptive normal birth was discussed. Some basic ideas were imposed to prevent problems and hopefully save lives. First was the principle of not being alone, but always having another woman present during the birth. It was suggested that this woman be specialized in birth and the problems associated with birth so would recognize problems as they arise. Immediately several requested to be that woman, and receive training.

Secondly, they were encouraged to maintain cleanliness during the birth by having clean water available for washing. They were also encouraged if possible to have soap. The women believed that their husbands could get this for them. Using soap and water to cleanse the mother, cleanse her hands, and anyone's hands that was aiding her could reduce infection.

Finally, the women were encouraged to not use rocks to cut the cord and most importantly, to use some grass or rope to tie off the cord first. In addition, to ask for their husband's "flint" or knife to be available to cut the cord after it was tied. They were to clean the knife with soap and water first. We discussed that infection could be one of the causes of death among the mothers and babies simply by using rocks to cut the cord. We also discussed that bleeding could cause death from the cord not being tied off first prior to cutting. The bleeding could come from the baby and the mother. Therefore, tying the cord must occur.

The men and women sat is awe listening. They understood that these very basic ideas could potentially save the lives of the women in the village. Many were so happy they began to cry. The sun began to set so the classroom ended for the day.

The next day we continued our clinic and made jokes about showers, warm baths and using a toilet that flushed. Every day in the clinic, we had the one on one opportunity to reinforce the teaching on normal childbirth and women's bodies. Daily, my tortilla skills improved, sort of.

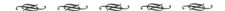

"Happy is the man who finds wisdom, And the man who gains understanding;" Proverbs 3:13

This experience in the mountains was profound to me. I had gained more wisdom and insight about God's people during this time. I had also learned the value of understanding culture. All people are part of God's plan, and He gave us so much knowledge to share with them. The Mexican Tarahumara gained understanding of pregnancy and birth and I gained much wisdom.

I returned home from this outreach changed. I knew my distinct purpose in life and the trek God had given me in preparation for times such as this. God showed me during the outreach that despite my own personal discomfort, lack of knowledge and wisdom, HE had a plan.

I left Mexico challenged and hungry to use more of my talents with His people on earth. I felt the call to action. I knew that all I needed to do now was walk in faith, and God will guide me. I knew also that I was about to embark into unchartered areas, and provide health care to as many people as I could reach. I new I had opened a new chapter in my life, and the lives of those I meet. Had I know then, what I know now, I probably would not have stepped out in faith to start a medical mission's organization. I am glad I did.

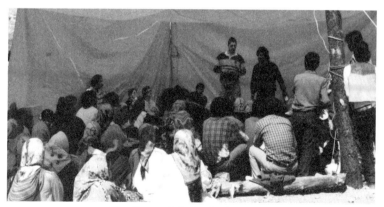

Our "mountain top" classroom.

Perhaps Tonight

"Bulat, Bulat" she stood peering out the large multi-paned empty window looking down on her husband. Large billowing snowflakes silently drifted from the dark wintery sky as the temperatures plummeted well below freezing. Icicles gallantly decorated the eaves and soffits of the building stretching to reach the ground without fracture. Misty fog loomed in the gardens while the warm breath of a young bride formed into a crystal tapestry on the window where she stood. Her eyes frantically searched the ground below for her true love. Just to capture a glimpse of his smile, she thought. It was seven o'clock, he must be somewhere she searched, "this is our time" she murmured, as tears begin to well in her eyes her hands stretched to grasp the cold window, as if the window alone would bring forth her love. "Bulat Bulat where are you"? Now, forty weeks pregnant, Natasha awaits the birth of her first child.

Bulat, a strong young Tartar man, braved the fury of winter's worst storms in hopes of getting a glimpse of his bride. "Perhaps tonight," he said as he wondered if she would be holding the baby that night. They planned prior to her admission to meet at seven o'clock every night. "Just to see her face" he knew then everything would be ok. He didn't miss a night, despite the cold blustery weather of Russia. He stood outside the gates of the hospital and peered up to see her face once again. Their eyes met.

The massive cement hospital empowered the ground it stood on. Stretching endlessly, with very few doors, the colossal facility enslaved its inhabitants as a prison incarcerates a criminal. Infinite cold blocks, repeatedly stacked uniformly one upon another, giving way to only a few mere windows. Empty windows, erect as a band of brothers, in an unbroken pattern of lineage scaled the outer wall, never changing all the same. The colossal structure stood as tall as it was wide, forging the oatmeal sky in massive authority while plummeting well beneath the frozen ground. The hospital held captive mothers and babies.

Natasha had been hospitalized for almost two weeks now, waiting to give birth. Her room was large. The tall walls extended high between the pale green tiled floor and the empty ceiling. Block after block her temporary home of whitewashed cement and empty windows plainly comforted her. No curtains, pictures, clocks or photos gave color or definition to the massive walls. The outside wall pelted with windows brought in the only light. Ten beds lined the inside wall. Some had cribs next to them and some did not. Every bed had a small straw stuffed mattress, two sheets and a wool blanket, nothing more nothing less. Each bed had one occupant, some waiting to give birth and others who had given birth. Personal items neatly stacked under the beds of their owners. Small sachets stuffed with a new baby blanket also neatly placed under each bed awaiting the new baby. Women labored here. Women recovered here. Women waited here.

Natasha came to the hospital under the instruction of her doctor. Admitted prior to the birth of her baby, her doctor instructed her as he did her mother, "it is important to keep you isolated from your family, friends, and the illnesses of our society prior to the birth of your baby, we don't want complications." She understood this isolation, from the world of disease, bacteria and death, was developed to protect her and her baby, her mother did it so should she. "Only for a short time" she was instructed, then after the baby was born and a week old and there were no complications she could go home. Confidently she agreed to go to the hospital and wait.

Natasha's eyes met Bulat's. A sigh of relief entered her lungs as she motioned to him that indeed she was still pregnant. They waved, longed to touch and hold each other once again but feared that he could present disease to her or the baby. He did not consider approaching her.

He carried a basket for her. Covered in cloth, Bulat scurried to the building to deliver the basket to his bride. Her mother had prepared a healthy portion of ham, potatoes, greens and dried fish for her to eat. His quick pace was halted by the hospital police. They would deliver the basket. The aroma of fresh baked bread filled the room as the evening guard peered beneath the blanket. His nose taunted him to try just one piece of the warm bread. It melted in his mouth as Bulat angrily scorned him. "Deliver the basket to my wife" Bulat demanded, "do not eat her food, I will bring you your portion tomorrow." After much confrontation the guard agreed to have the food delivered, Bulat was escorted outside. Ice pellets dropped from the sky, adjusting his hat and collar Bulat waited.

The basket contained food for Natasha. There were no cafeterias or food service in the hospital. Every patient in the hospital needed family members to bring them food daily. The families were not allowed into the hospital only to drop off the food and leave again. Sadly, those who do not have family are left to beg for food from other patients. However, several nurses would often leave portions for them from their own food or leftover patients. Natasha's family provided healthy portions of food, knowing that others may also need some. The basket arrived to Natasha about one hour later. Bulat, nearly frozen, waved goodbye to his bride and left for home.

Moaning heard in a nearby bed, another woman and roommate was in labor. This happened almost every other night, someone would be in labor, or others up with a crying baby. Sleep was difficult for Natasha when another woman was in labor. She feared what was happening and the pain she too would soon endure yet still welcomed her day to come quickly. "Just to hold the baby," she smiled, "and to be with Bulat again soon." The woman tonight moaned rhythmically and continuously and cried out for help, no one came. Natasha and a few other women stood at her bed stroking her hair, sometimes holding her hand. More experienced women would encourage her and offer suggestions to aid in comfort. The night passed, the moaning did not. Nurses would come in from time to time, stand and watch and then leave. Natasha stayed.

Moaning, moaning, it became louder and closer. The nurses returned to the room intuitively as if they knew somehow that the birth was eminent. They would discuss the situation, check the woman and leave. Soon they returned to her bedside and summoned her to walk down the hallway into another place. It was silent, the moans were gone. Natasha laid her head down on her pillow while listening to the muffled screams of her new friend beyond closed doors. It wasn't long before the screams stopped. Silence penetrated the halls. Natasha fell into a deep exhausted sleep as her baby danced in her belly. Instinctively she rubbed her baby.

Hours passed, and new her friend returned to her small bed. Natasha awakened and sat up in bed ready to discuss and learn the details of her birth and her new baby. Something was different. Her arms were empty, without child. There was no response. Natasha sat quietly as the nurses assisted her friend to bed. She lay motionless in the bed as if life had drained from her body. "What happened" inquired Natasha, "where is the baby" she asked quietly. One nurse coldly turned to her and with piercing eyes stated, "The baby is dead, and your friend will be too if she doesn't rest." Natasha so badly wanted to reach out and hold her friend closely, dearly and comfort her pain. But, the pain struck her own womb deeply, "no don't let my baby die." Fear gripped Natasha by the throat, her lungs filled with air and her breathing increased as a car goes into over drive. Her hands and feet became numb and began to tingle. Fear overcame her as she slumped to the floor in a cold sweat. Time passed.

Natasha awoke, her room unchanged, now in her bed. As if time stood still she instinctively jumped to her feet and massaged her belly "yes" she thought, "my baby is still alive within me." Searching the room for her friend, she found her lying motionless in her bed. Blankets pulled high over her body, as if to hide her barren womb. Natasha approached the bed, pulled back the blankets, and nestled closely behind her friend. Reaching her arms around the woman's shoulders she pulled her friend in closely towards her bosom and the warmth of her body. No words were spoken, only the swift beating of one mother's heart to fill another mother's emptiness could be heard. Evening came.

Natasha jumped to her feet realizing that it was time to meet Bulat. Sprinting to the window she frantically searched for him, no where could he be seen. The frigid winter air bellowed through the open window as Natasha stretched to search every aspect of the gardens outside. "Bulat!" she cried out "Bulat!" secretly hoping he could hear her. "I just want to tell him what happened," her eyes still searching, "I need to see you my love." Looking back at her bed she saw her basket, replenished and full of food. Time had passed as she comforted her friend, it was midnight, Bulat had come and went hours prior. Exhausted, Natasha returned to her bed. She did not desire to eat, only to reside in the comfort of her active baby and to trust in God to keep her baby alive.

The sun shone brightly as the clouds dispersed and the teal blue sky was vividly seen through the lanky windows. Warmth filled the room with the chatter of women and the cries of newborn babies. Natasha, however, chose to stay in bed. Pain and discomfort towards the loss of a baby filled her heart. She told the women companions she was too sick to get up today. Her cries changed to moans and soon began to fill the room. Her friend, now at her side, to comfort her, cried with her. Natasha was in labor.

Natasha was afraid. She feared the death of her baby. She feared the pain she was enduring. She deeply wanted Bulat to be with her, or her mother. She found comfort in the women around her, and her friend whose arms were empty.

The pains became rhythmic. She knew when they were coming and tried to be prepared by not getting tense or tight. She had seen other women go through this and knew it was better to relax than to fight it. The women surrounded her with comfort and suggestions. The pain came closer and closer together. Natasha felt the grip of fear choking her as if she were drowning in a river full of rocks and rapids. She wanted to fight for her breath for her life, but her friends told her to ride the waves out. Then she pictured the river coming to a bend and she could float like a smooth sailing raft. She found rest, for a short time, then again, she would go through the rocks and rapids, searching for the bend to give her peace, it came. "How much longer can I last?" she asked her friends. "You will last," they replied, "your baby is waiting for you at the end of the rapids, you will get there soon." She tried to picture her baby at the end of the river.

The nurses came in and checked her. They told her it was time, and she could walk with them down the hall. She tried to get up but could not, her body was tight with pain and tension. "How can I walk?!" she pleaded. "You must," the nurse replied, "it is time."

Natasha walked down the long hall. One foot in front of the other, grasping the bar on the side with each step became her pathway. Warm liquid ran from her body, down her legs, onto the floor. She looked down, it was green, fearfully she cried out "What is happening, what is this liquid, is my baby ok?" Tears began to flow from her eyes and down her cheeks. "Keeping walking," said the nurse sternly. "I can't," she replied "I can't." Without much a due the nurse reached out and took Natasha by the arm as a guard escorts a prisoner and stated, "You must." Natasha approached the delivery room.

Turning the corner, she entered the room. The smell of chemicals filled her burning nostrils as she took each breath. The odor was so strong she felt the welling urge in her stomach encouraging her to vomit. Following instructions, she sat down in an unusual shaped chair. The chair was mustard colored and had a stately high back as if made for a queen. Yet there was not a bottom to sit on only partial areas for each leg jutted out on each side. Once seated, straps draped as a seat belt in a car quickly secured her body. Arms extended out to her sides were also strapped to a board of sorts and legs anchored to the chair. The chair lifted off the floor and then tilted back. Pains continued to come and breathing changed to grunting. "Is my baby ok?" she murmured. No one responded as she watched a fluttering of people enter the room. "Is my baby ok!" she cried, while a black mask covered her face.

Natasha awoke. Rubbing her belly, she found it empty giving her a start. Sitting erect in bed she loudly cried out "Where is my baby, Where is my baby!" Jumping to her feet her body stopped by the firm grip on her shoulders from a nurse as she attempted to lower her back into her bed. "Your baby girl is fine," she stated, "now lay back down, you must rest." "A girl? Where is she, I must she her," Natasha wept.

"There was a complication, you must wait." The nurse stated, "Your baby is in isolation."

"What is isolation!" she cried out again. "I need to see my baby!"

The force from the nurse lowered Natasha back into her bed, as she laid down the nurse said again "Your baby is fine, now lay back down."

Natasha could no longer hold back her fears and tears as she wept freely. Head pounding and heart crying she looked at the clock. It was nearly seven o'clock, I must tell Bulat. Instinctively leaping to the floor she lunged for the window hoping to see Bulat. The nurse had no strength to battle the strength a heart has for a loved one. The window flew open as the room filled with winter air and snow flurried around Natasha, Bulat was standing just below as planned waiting to see his bride for it had been over two days. "Bulat!" she cried out, "I had the baby, but she is gone, I do not know where, I do not know why, she is here somewhere, please help me find her, oh Bulat please help me!" The nurse halted her words and she pulled Natasha back into bed and firmly locked the window.

Bulat stood in the snow covered garden paralyzed by her words, wanting desperately to hold his wife and see their baby. Without forethought, he snapped, running into the hospital, bursting through the gates, throwing back the doors Bulat sought out his family. Halted immediately by guards holding him back and threatening their weapons he retreated momentarily. Angrily he demanded to see his wife and baby. The guards refused his request and threatened him again with weapons drawn now calling for police. Bulat did his best to calm himself and again asked for their assistance regarding his family, they again denied him information or entrance further into the facility. Bulat offered a generous sum of money to the guards for information about his wife. The guards happily accepted the generous offer of money and went to inquire about his wife Natasha. They sent for the courier of baskets to request of the nurse's information about Natasha. The courier took the basket and quickly began the flight of stairs to the floor she resided. Just then, the metal doors of the hospital entrance burst open bringing forth an influx of police officers. The encroachment of force coupled with the crippling sound of handcuffs pierced the air as Bulat was restrained. The hospital guards smirked while counting their financial reward and stood back watching as Bulat was bound and forcefully removed from the hospital. Doors slamming and locks clacking, the hospital was secured. Bulat was then escorted to the police station for disorderly conducted and was detained.

Natasha fell into depression. Refusing to eat or drink she lay motionless in her bed. Bulat no longer came to the window. Enduring the grief, she painfully watched other mothers feed, hold, and care for their babies. Her mind and body longed for her baby. Breasts swelling and belly cramping she wanted so badly to fill her arms with a baby, her baby. "Where is my baby?" she asked everyone who entered the room. Now, out of fear themselves and the uncomfortable feeling of hopelessness, no one would approach her bed, she feared the worst.

Day three, Natasha was awakened by rustling in the room and an entourage of people surrounding her bed including the nurses. "Wake up, Wake up," she heard familiar voices calling her. Reluctantly, she removed the woolen blanket from her head and allowed the bright sunlight to waken her swollen eyes. Scanning the room, she saw all her roommates standing over her. "Leave me alone!" she scowled and began to retreat beneath the covers when her eyes locked onto a nurse standing at her feet, smiling so big one could count her teeth, cuddling a baby tightly bound in a familiar blanket. "It's your baby!" they all shouted. Natasha immediately sat up and began to question the nurse "What do you mean, my baby, I thought, something was wrong, something happened!" she began to cry. "What, my baby?" She quickly looked under her bed to find the sachet holding a baby blanket and cloths missing, they were gone. Looking again at the baby, and the blanket, impulsively she reached out for the baby. She began to weep uncontrollably. Her friends hugged her and helped her embrace the baby for the first time. Her tears turned to sobs as she welcomed her baby in her arms for the first time. Hello baby!

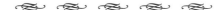

Natasha's story reminds me of the Scripture found in John 16:21:

"A woman, when she is in labor, has sorrow because her hour has come; but as soon as she has given birth to the child, she no longer remembers the anguish, for joy that a human being has been born into the world."

Natasha & Bulat served as Russian interpreters for me during several outreaches in their homeland. They were reunited two days later as Natasha was discharged from the hospital with her newborn baby. Both of them had the opportunity to visit the USA and stay at our home. During their time here we visited several U.S. hospital labor and delivery suites and birth centers. Natasha recalls that the birth of her first baby was very terrifying and she never learned why her baby was isolated from her. We had the wonderful opportunity to host Natasha and Bulat in our home for several weeks in the U.S. We openly talked about birth and invited them to tour several birth centers, hospitals and birthing options in America. During their visit to the U.S., they conceived baby number two and Natasha did not fear this birth as she did the first time.

Happily, she gave birth to her second daughter in Russia with Bulat present. She opened wrote to me in a letter, "This birth happened under different circumstances." Natasha wrote, "I love my country and understand they are trying to protect me and my baby from disease. However, birth is not a disease but it happens to most women. Our women in Russia do not talk about giving birth. Our mothers teach us to work not give birth.

I know so much more now, and understand that my biggest fear was the fear itself." Natasha also shared she plans to teach her daughters and encourage other mothers to talk to their daughters about birth. In closing she wrote, "Women need to share with each other so they do not experience the fear she had, so they can enjoy their babies and understand that birth is normal."

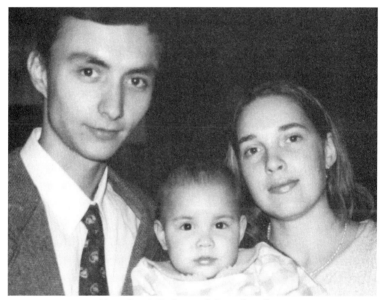

Natasha & Bulat and their daughter.

Then You Came

Despite the sinking sun, sweat poured from our heated bodies. We were a small team of American midwives in south central China teaching other midwives, doctors and nurses about childbirth. This area had never before received American visitors, so we drew quite a crowd. It was fun, teaching in the mornings and then consulting with the Chinese providers in the afternoon. The only drawback was the intense heat. Sleep was difficult, because our rooms had no fans or windows—just an entrance. Because there was no circulation of the hot humid air, I took a shower before bed to cool my body—no hot water, but inviting mountain spring water.

Our last night in the country I slept well, but woke suddenly to the screams of one of our team members. A Chinese nurse had touched Ginger's shoulder to wake her, eliciting from her a blood-curdling scream. I bolted from my bunk, jumped to the floor and ran out into the hall. As the screams continued, my heart pounded. I was not sure if I should run, scream or hide myself. Nevertheless, I stood in the doorway of Ginger's room and shouted, "Are you okay?"

Ginger and Denise both replied, "Yes, yes, oh my goodness, yes."

"I'm so sorry I scared you, Ginger said. "I guess I just reacted to someone touching me."

Then we saw the Chinese nurse standing near the bed. I think she was more scared than we were. She motioned for us to hurry and follow her as we were being requested to help with a birth. It was about three o'clock in the morning.

Stumbling around, we grabbed our shoes, jumped into scrubs and followed the nurse into the hospital. Turning into the maternity unit, I heard the muffled sounds of people working. The delivery room was well lit, the smell of formalin and alcohol penetrated the air. On the delivery table lay a young Chinese woman who had just delivered a baby. Her husband fretfully held her head while the birth attendant stitched a large episiotomy.

We hurriedly entered the room, and I scanned the scene, wondering why they woke us up. The baby was already born. What was happening?

The nurse summoned us to the cabinet. Under a quilted blanket lay a flaccid baby girl.

Oh, my God, I thought, as I instinctively moved into an ER Nurse mode. Grasping the baby, my fingers palpated the umbilical cord. Yes, there was a weak pulse. Without even a thought, I started giving orders and verbally stating my assessment aloud, as if all present could understand English.

"Baby has a pulse of eighty," I said is a commanding voice. Continuing my assessment, I noted she was not breathing.

"Ambu-bag. Is there an Ambu-bag?" I looked up at my team members who were still half-asleep and moving into action. Obviously, there were not any Ambu-bags around, but my mind was still in USA ER mentality.

Turning back towards the baby, I gently lifted her head back, slid the towel that covered her under her shoulders and gave her two short breaths. My mouth to her nose and mouth. Two breaths. Yes, I saw her chest rise and fall. She then took her own breath. Her body felt cold and lifeless on the hard cabinet.

She whimpered. "Yes, yes. Come on baby, you can do it."

A weak cry, but to me, it was a cry. I was thrilled, but could not elicit more of a response. "Come on baby." I used that same towel to rub her back and head. "Come on baby, I need some more cries from you."

Her heart rate was increasing, slightly over 100, and she moved one of her arms, just a little. Ginger asked, "When was she born? What problems happened? Any infection?"

But no one answered. We realized the Chinese had called us to help, but we did not have our interpreter with us. We were clueless as to why we were awakened for this baby, and why she was lying on the counter without anyone attending to her, lifeless.

I continued to assess the baby. Her heart rate was stronger, and I did not hear any murmurs. She appeared normal; all fingers and toes, normal in appearance. She had breath sounds on both sides of her lungs and normal lung sounds.

"What do you think?" I said to my friends. "I'm not sure what to do."

We verbally followed the neonatal resuscitation algorithm to see if we had missed anything. What to do next? Our voices scanned the mental algorithm. Flexing her arms and legs, this newborn baby was making great attempts at maintaining life. Her heart rate was 130, and she was breathing on her own at about forty breaths per minute.

"She just needed a jump start," I said. "What happened anyway?" I looked around the room, as if someone would answer my question. My eyes locked on to those of the young mother, and knowing she did not understand English, I smiled at her and gave her a "thumbs up" sign. She smiled, and then began to cry.

The baby's cry remained weak. Her pulse was strong, respirations normal, but her legs hung limp with the color not as pink as we would like. One of our team members, Sue an awesome pediatric nurse, recommended we initiate an IV and perhaps some glucose to stimulate her. We tried to communicate this to the Chinese nurse who had summoned our help. She seemed to understand, but wanted us to go with her to the pediatric ward. Should we move this baby away from the mother? We decided to abide by the request and go to pediatrics. With no formal transport system to move the baby to pediatrics, I picked her up, gently cuddled her little body into a fetal position, lifted my own shirt, and placed her next to my skin. Eyebrows in the room rose. I was sure the Chinese nurse thought I was either trying to take the baby or I was just plain crazy.

One of our American team members said, "What are you doing, Cathy?"

"Keeping her warm." I replied while gently caressing the tiny baby.

Out the delivery room, around several corners, down halls then up a flight of stairs, I carried this baby, still under my shirt. It was awkward. I had nothing on but scrubs, no underwear or t-shirt, and lifting my shirt to view her meant I was more exposed. In addition, I really could not assess the baby while she was bundled up in my shirt. I wanted so badly to look at her, to ensure she was still breathing and getting pink. I only knew that her body was cold.

The room in pediatrics was empty except for a small crib pushed up against the wall. Whitewashed walls, no pictures, no clock or chairs, only the crib lined the vacant wall. Placing the baby in the crib, I reassessed her.

"Pulse 130." I said. "Respiration's fifty-two." Her color, flexion and tone remained unchanged.

Chinese nurses entered the room and presented us with glass IV bottles, tubing and IV catheters. Yippee, I thought, while reaching for the supplies. I smiled at the nurses, decked out in white uniforms and caps. Their smiles and sparkling eyes illuminated the room.

I was thrilled that we were actually communicating, despite our language barrier. One of our team members performed theatrical sign language that we needed IV fluids. She demonstrated how to put an IV in, cried that it hurt, and used tubing. Her mime demonstration was exactly what we needed. The nurses liked her and understood.

"Good work, Denise," I said.

Sue assembled the IV supplies and prepared to start an IV. Then she said, "Cathy, these bottles are warm."

"What? The bottles are warm?"

Before I could grasp one, the Chinese nurses took the baby and gently placed two bottles on each side of her in a large blanket. They rolled her, tucked the blanket and swaddled her into a huge package. Snuggled around those bottles, the newborn opened her eyes and looked around for more. Her body temperature slowly warmed.

Apparently, when the nurse in the delivery unit saw me place the baby under my shirt, she sent someone to notify the pediatric nurses to heat the bottles. Since there were no blanket warmers or microwaves in the building, they used a charcoal cook stove to heat the bottles.

Sue, our pediatric nurse, inserted a small IV into the baby's tiny hand. The baby winced and cried. Soon she was wailing. The solid cry of this newborn was like music at an outdoor concert. We were thrilled. "Yes, yes, yes," I shouted. "Thank you, God."

Not really knowing the entire birth history, we began to discuss the possibilities. The sun was now up, and our stomachs growled. The Chinese nurses assumed care of the newborn. We encouraged the nurses to take the baby to the mother as soon as possible for breastfeeding. Watching our visual demonstration again, they nodded their heads, smiled, and took the baby from us to the waiting mother.

Our interpreter met us for breakfast. We sat at an outdoor restaurant in the hospital compound and recited the story. Our animation and excitement drew a Chinese crowd of curious onlookers who wanted to understand why these American foreigners were so excited. We sat at a round table, ate pork dumplings and rice, and cackled like hens in a brooder house. Our translator did her best to answer our questions. Our excitement fueled from the adrenalin of the night.

Our final rounds at the hospital were hard, leaving the Chinese medical team we had come to know so well. Our last client was the mother who had just given birth. She now held her baby, who was breastfeeding like a trooper, and doing all the normal baby things like pooping and peeing. We all stood around her bed to and listened to her story, of course with the aid of our interpreter.

"I met you yesterday, when I came to the prenatal clinic," she stated. "You all were so kind and gentle with me." When my labor started, I asked the attendant to call for you, but they did not want to wake you because you were departing today. They said they wanted you to rest well before your long journey."

The tone of her voice was fearful, so our translator did her best to tell us what she said. I sat next to the mother on the bed and listened.

"My baby was born, and she did not cry. They took her over there and laid her down. She was moving, but not crying so I cried out for you.

"I shouted, 'Americans, Americans,' in hopes, you would hear me. I knew you would help my baby. My husband then also demanded they call for the Americans. I kept shouting for you even though they told me to be quiet. The attendant finally summoned you to come. Meanwhile the baby lay on the cabinet, covered with the blanket. I continued to cry for my baby. Then you came."

While writing this story I could not help but feel as if the Hebrew midwives in the Bible, were challenged with a similar trial. The difference is only the country. Both situations the midwives are encouraged to partake in a form of infanticide or mercy killing for the sake of the governmental sanction. In the Bible, the midwives were encouraged to kill all the baby boys once they were born, and throw the in the river. Read Exodus 1:15-16:

"The king of Egypt said to the Hebrew midwives, whose names were Shiphrah and Puah, 'When you help the Hebrew women in childbirth and observe them on the delivery stool, if it is a boy, kill him; but if it is a girl, let her live.'"

Health care providers are often encouraged by government, peer pressure, and even pressure of "freedom of choice" to perform procedures that do not fall in line with God's law. The Hebrew midwives feared God and did not adhere to the governmental call upon them to kill baby boys. Rather, some hid the babies as in the case of Moses.

China adopted a policy in the 1970s, restricting most Chinese households to only one child. This form of human family planning developed by the government was in an effort to control the fast growing population, aid the economy and protect the environment from the rapid growth. The policy also enforced fines on families who had more than one child, or those who had female babies. Government-mandated abortions were forced on women who became pregnant and already had children. During our time in China, we noted that indeed many abortions are performed daily.

The government also reported a large decrease in female births over the next ten years. They noted a decrease in birth certificates being processed and well over 80 percent were of male children. They believed the control of the population was working.

Sadly, the decrease in female births attributed to infanticide, abortions, and stillbirth is on the rise. Infanticide is the homicide of a viable baby. Viability is determined after a baby passes twenty weeks gestation. Infanticide performed after birth is a way of decreasing viability. Late term abortions are the argumentative version of infanticide where the mother is induced into labor, the baby's head is born and the baby's life is stopped prior to the birth of the body. The various means of late term abortion are too graphic to record. After delivery of the body, the baby is recorded as a stillbirth.

Late term abortion, also deemed as selective-sex abortion, is reported in many Chinese provinces. Ultrasound is used to determine the gender of a baby. If the unborn baby is identified as a girl, the woman undergoes a late term abortion, sex-selective abortion, based on gender criteria alone.

Many baby girls are not attended to at birth. Once they are born, no one dries them, stimulates them, or clears their airways. They are laid aside to die. Baby boys are attended to immediately after birth, because they bring honor and status to the family. The family lineage continues through the seed of the male child. The pressure on each woman to give birth to a son is greater than any pressure perceived in the country.

On this particular day, this mother used her knowledge and foresight to call for help. She knew involving foreigners could cost her more than just her baby's life; it could cause much trouble for her family. She knew she could go to prison for involving foreigners, especially if they reported to the press that the Chinese were doing something wrong. Calling for help was dangerous; especially help from an American, but her voice was heard.

The cries from women for their babies pierce our hearts and must be heard. Ginger eloquently stated as we departed, "This was a demonstration of a life worth saving."

On this day, one baby girl lived.

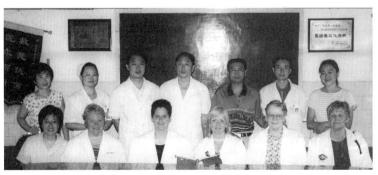

Our team.

I'm Spittin'

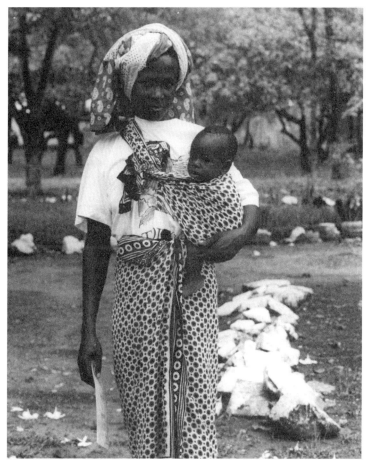

Kenyan mother and baby.

Trekking from village to village, our team of health care providers offered free health care consultations, examinations and medications to many families in need. We were in the heart of East African food, culture and language challenges. After four short weeks in the country, our flexible team had transformed every type of setting into a clinic arena. Under trees, inside homes, along the banks of a river and within the walls of vacant buildings, almost any area became a makeshift clinical setting.

Over 3,000 people received healing from diseases and illnesses. Before the sun peeked over the horizon, families arrived to secure a place in line. They waited hours for a brief consultation from a health care provider—a precious consultation because the health care providers were Americans.

Tired, dusty feet revealed a life of endurance and hard labor, as each African hoped for relief from various ailments. Many had never seen an actual trained health care provider, let alone an American. Anxiously they waited, their faces revealing true desperation and the hardship of a life of daily survival.

Babies swaddled with colorful fabrics snuggled securely to the mother's back. Toddlers hid within their mother's Katanga, fearful that the foreigners might prey upon them.

Katangas, worn by women throughout the continent of Africa, have become a signature of African culture. They consist of a long fabric cloth that wraps around the woman's waist and ties or tucks in securely so as not to fall off. It covers the entire length of the legs. Many Katangas reveal political statements or a common greeting from the country of service. They are given out freely during campaigns so that the women model them. Like human billboards, these women adorn their heads with matching cloths. Few wear shoes.

Our clinic was full and busy with a commonality of complaints. As if a virus had impacted the village, during each consultation the women stated, "I'm spittin' Ms. Cathy." Many carried a cup or a bowl to use as a spittoon.

Why would so many women complain of "spitting?" This most unusual and relatively common "chief complaint" surprised and puzzled our team. Was it the food they ate that caused this symptom or maybe a sore throat infestation like strep?

We huddled to discuss the cause. Our African friends laughed as they revealed the root of the problem to us American Mazungu's. This unrelenting and common presentation by the African women was a sign of pregnancy, called Ptyalism in the medical world, and a common thread in this African community.

The women, who presented with the complaint of spitting, wanted a prenatal evaluation. We were thrilled to offer examinations and prenatal vitamins for the duration of their pregnancies. However, the thought of so many women with ptyalism seemed overwhelming. Was this some type of genetic link?

Frequent salivation, or "spittin'", was the sign of pregnancy to many women in this village area, because the more common signs of pregnancy often went undetected. These women breastfed their babies for at least two years, which masked a "missed period" and or possible "breast tenderness" as a sign of pregnancy. Excessive saliva meant the woman was pregnant.

Research reveals that ptyalism only affects a small population of women. Unfortunately, there is limited information as to why some women suffer with it and others do not. Those who deal with ptyalism are rarely relieved of their condition until after the birth of the baby.

Some authors have suggested that the excessive salivation may be a result of unswallowed saliva. When women experience nausea and vomiting known as "morning sickness," they produce more saliva. Those who do not swallow the excess, spit it out. Other authors claim it is a disease state called "Hyperemesis gravidarum."

Hyperemesis gravidarum, defined as profound nausea of pregnancy, is a possible precursor of ptyalism. Increased salivation is linked to heartburn, which is another common complaint women have in pregnancy. None of the women coming to our clinic complained of heartburn, however, most carried a cup to spit their excessive salvia into. I could not help but wonder if these African women were suffering from the Hyperemesis gravidarum.

We noted that many of the women did indeed swallow some of their saliva. Normal production of saliva is about 700ml per day and goes unnoticed by most people, because it is swallowed. These women could easily expel about 200ml (about one cup) of saliva per visit. That in itself seemed like a lot of saliva, whether they swallowed it or not.

We considered the possibility of a genetic predisposition or thyroid disease as a causative factor. Unfortunately, we were not equipped to run a CBC or a TSH. When I returned to the U.S., none of my colleagues had seen many women with the condition of Ptyalism nor did they suggest any treatment regimens.

I have learned that other women from various countries of the world also suffer from Ptyalism. However, I personally have found that women who are of African descent present with this complaint than from any other continent, specifically the Sub-Saharan countries of Africa.

I asked these African women and those who had immigrated to the U.S., "What did you do to relieve your symptoms?"

Amazingly, I learned that they found relief from the Kola Nut.

The Kola Nut, also called Guru, is indigenous to Western Africa, primarily Nigeria, Congo, Sierra Leone and Guinea. It is also found in Jamaica, due to transplantation for the purposes of commerce and trade. The kola Nut tree is about forty to sixty feet high, with thick green bark. The nut or fruit of the tree may be a purple or white oblong seed about two to three cm long. The nut is best for tea. However, many Africans add it to meals or in its raw form they chew on it and suck it for the relief of a variety of symptoms. Many shared relief from upset stomach or digestive problems including diarrhea, eructation or vomiting and difficulty swallowing—even during pregnancy. In addition, many claimed great relief from depression, anxiety and migraine headaches.

While working in Africa, I learned about the different varieties of Kola Nut in the market. I purchased both the white and purple seeds and took them to the midwives I worked with in the different countries. Initially, they laughed at me for buying the nut they called guru, because they had it readily available and they believed I had spent my money needlessly. They shared with me exactly how they used this nut.

African midwives claimed that shaving a small piece from the nut and placing this piece along the gum and lower teeth was one of the best remedies for excessive spitting or any upset stomach . They shared many different uses, including the uplifting of spirits and reducing fatigue. During our conversation, the Kola Nut was thinly sliced and shared with everyone to enjoy, including me.

The action of the Kola Nut is similar to coffee and cocoa, with a slightly different presentation of caffeine and theobromine.

It appears to exert a tonic influence, improving digestion by increasing secretion or by acting upon the circular fibers of the stomach. It is not surprising then that it could influence the production and movement of excessive saliva, thereby decreasing the symptoms many African women encounter during pregnancy. Taken in small amounts sublingually, many traditional midwives and Africa women use this great resource to reduce excessive salivation or "spittin'".

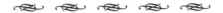

While working in Kenya during this outreach, I am reminded of the Bible verse in Isaiah 52:7. I learned so much in Kenya. The many miles these women trekked just to see our team, brought us so much joy. Their feet walked in faith.

"How beautiful upon the mountains are the feet of him who brings good news, Who proclaims peace, Who brings glad tidings of good things, Who proclaims salvation, Who says to Zion, 'Your God reigns!'"

God's kingdom does reign here on earth. We can learn so much from other nations, cultures and women. Unfortunately, in the U.S., it is hard to find fresh Kola Nut, but the extract can be found in herbal product stores. Pharmacologically, it is recommended that some ptyalism can be reduced with the use of traditional medications such as REGLAN or metoclopramide which increases gastric motility. However, over the last several years I have found great success using alternative treatments such as the Kola Nut. The Africans understand the presentation well, and know the best remedy. We health care providers have now learned an alternative treatment for ptyalism.

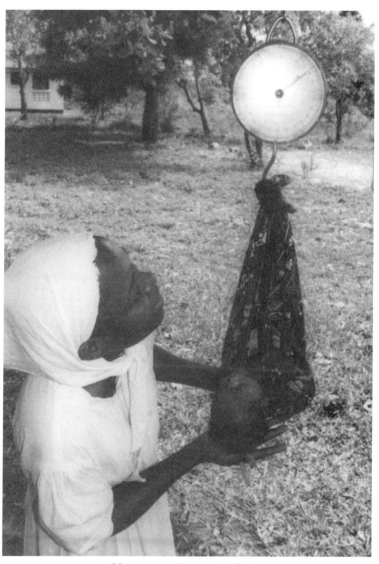

Margaret, a Kenyan Midwife.

Where Will I Go To Have My Baby?

January 12, 2010, earmarked one of the world's worst disasters. A devastating earthquake in Haiti, measuring a 7.0 magnitude, violently rocked the cities of Port au Prince and Jacmel killing 250,000, injuring 300,000 and leaving well over 1,000,000 people homeless. The cry for help echoed from this small developing nation for aid, medical care and "to find their dead and rescue any injured." The cry pierced the ears and hearts of every nation around the globe. Rescuers mobilized as the aftershocks continued for another ten days, leveling many remaining structures and buildings and stalling rescue efforts for any possible survivors. Cries of pain and agony were heard across the globe and the world responded.

Americans immediately answered the call. Organizations such as Missionary Aviation Flights sent planes full of rescuers and health care providers into Haiti. Time was of the essence. Survivors hung on to hope. Many lost limbs or gave birth in the middle of the rubble. Rescuers had limited access to the country, due to the extensive damage. Planes could not land in Haiti without daylight due to the damaged airport. There was no electricity; no accessible terminal and only one working runway open for safe landings.

Our plane boarded with surgeons, nurse practitioners, internists, nurses, and me—the experienced midwife in childbirth. We approached Port au Prince. The view was unforgettable.

I gazed out of the plane's window and saw buildings whose exterior resembled a stack of pancakes. Helicopters appeared from the midst of the rubble, lifting rescue baskets. Military aircraft surrounded us, gathering the wounded. As our plane taxied to the temporary terminal, we silently observed the hundreds of relief workers already in place.

Bases of United Nations personnel lined the airport tarmac and runways. National flags from working nations flew high above their camps. These flags, gently blowing in the Haitian breeze, represented several countries I did not recognize. It was breathtaking to view the many base camps from countries such as South Korea, Mexico, Japan, Germany, Canada and many more. My eyes welled with tears as trucks and jeeps carried victims to other planes.

I quietly prayed, "May God bless these workers and those whom they are caring for."

Entering the temporary terminal, we were met by immigration officials and departing relief workers. Their dirty bodies and torn clothes highlighted their mission. Their faces depicted the difficult trials they had endured during the initial rescue efforts, some smiling; others solemn. They boarded our empty plane, certainly anxious for a warm shower and toothbrush while we were being processed into the country. Carrying my backpack and bedroll, I shook hands with as many as I could and thanked them for their work. I could not help but wonder if I would be as strong as they had been.

The back of a truck became our transportation. As we rode through the city to our camp, we viewed the devastation. Fallen homes, schools, churches and stores were everywhere, including survivors who searched for the missing. We rode silently.

Arriving at our camp, we were debriefed about ongoing rescue efforts. Divided into teams, we prepared to depart to one of the many relief effort stations and work while sunlight was available. Our temporary home was a Christian School, amazingly untouched by the quake. The large enclosed area had several buildings; including a large schoolyard and soccer field. This became the mission base for the U.S. military and many other medical teams.

At least 100 health care providers camped in the area— French, Dutch, German, Swedish, and Japanese medical personnel, including several U.S. teams. Our base leaders were missionaries from the U.S. who grew up in Haiti. The day after the earthquake, they had returned to their "hometown" to help. Their eyes filled with tears as they saw me sitting among the team.

"Cathy," they shouted and sprinted toward me. "You came. I can't believe you came."

We embraced and to the amazement of the medical team, I was introduced by the two team leaders as their "midwife." Not long before, in Kansas City, I had delivered their wives' babies within months of each other. The wives had e-mailed me and asked me to come and help in Haiti. For a brief moment, I felt like a movie star!

I sat with these leaders and heard their plea for help. They tearfully shared that while they were removing rubble from a building, a woman survivor was believed to be in labor. The closest hospital had fallen in the earthquake. No health care providers were available and there was no transportation to get her to a medical team.

One of the men, Theo, promised to stay with this woman and help her. He had been present when his wife delivered their two young children. He comforted and encouraged the woman as she lay still on the sidewalk. He offered her water and attempted to keep her comfortable with a pillow he made from some nearby clothing.

"Her breathing was erratic, and her eyes were staring as if she wasn't really there," Theo said. "I knew her labor was progressing because her breathing changed and she started having contractions. She finally looked at me, sat up slightly and started to push.

"I did my best to help her, realizing she had broken bones and needed a lot of support," he added. His head dropped and he continued in a whisper. "She soon delivered a baby boy, but he never tried to breathe. He was dead."

After a long pause, Theo added, "Within a few minutes, the woman stopped breathing and died. I wanted so badly to help her."

"You did, Theo," I said. "You did."

The stress of the earthquake alone caused many women to go into labor. Sadly, many of them gave birth to pre-term or stillborn babies. Unfortunately, most babies were delivered by untrained birth attendants, on the streets of Haiti. Usually, this was someone who just wanted to help. Stories revealed, the Haitian Samaritan may have also unintentionally caused the woman's and her baby's death due to lack of knowledge, coupled with the earthquake trauma . They were trying to help.

Another woman gave birth amidst the rubble of a fallen building while her leg remained trapped. Soon after the delivery, the woman was rescued from the rubble but died due to blood loss. The need for trained midwives and health care providers mounted.

I sat with our two team leaders and listened to stories of the rescue efforts and medical dilemmas they had faced. I could see their hearts were tender in the midst of so much devastation. I knew then, why their wives had called me. They hoped, God willing, that maybe one life might be saved, and their work would be beneficial.

Our team divided and prepared to depart. Throwing my backpack on, I jumped into the back of the truck once again and headed out to work at one of the two epicenters, Carrefour. Just over a week had passed since the earthquake flattened the area. The smell of death and destruction still hung in the air. I searched for the box of surgical masks I had packed and was so glad I did.

My stomach is weak, and I easily get very nauseated and sometimes vomit at strong smells. I dropped wintergreen oil in the mask and snuggly placed it over my face, knowing the lingering smell of death and decay loomed over the city.

Driving through town, we witnessed firsthand the devastation the media had portrayed. The smell of decay and death lingered. I tried to gather strength for the work as I watched myriads of soldiers and health care workers aid the injured. Tent hospitals and clinics became overwhelmed with casualties, scores of wounded, and even more Haitians who only wanted shelter, food and water. We arrived at the stadium, now home to thousands of Haitians. The athletic grounds were covered with tents made from tarps held together by a single base pole and twine. These small tents lined up side by side to hold as many people as possible. These desperate people were hungry. They needed water and healthcare, and they quickly surrounded our truck.

I encouraged our team to wait. We needed to maintain order so as not to be mobbed. My experience had taught me that desperate people often resort to desperate measures. Slowly the crowd allowed our truck to advance. We moved toward the business office where we would set up our clinic. Scores of people reached for us, begging for food and water. Some tried to jump in the truck. Mothers offered their children to us, many still with open wounds, obvious fractures and debilitating injuries. Still advancing, we tried to avoid the people and maintain safety, but our truck came to an abrupt stop. The mob surrounded us. Fear began to creep in.

Within moments, the U.S. military surrounded our truck and walked alongside us. They demanded order from the crowd. They encouraged the people to stay back and allow us safe entry or they would turn us back. Their military demeanor, uniforms and weapons provided a level of expertise and command over the crowd. Once again, the mob settled, and order took place. I was so proud of our military, particularly this National Guard unit from North Carolina. They were well organized, took charge, and were very kind to everyone. U.S. forces seemed to be everywhere, organizing food and water and aiding medical teams so that they could do their jobs.

Our clinic mobilized into several stations: wounded, sick and others. It didn't take long for me to concentrate only on the pregnant women—so many pregnant women. Within a few days, I saw over 150 of them. The mothers were commonly suffering from post-traumatic stress and grave dehydration. The dehydration presentation was so profound; I could actually palpate toes of the babies on the abdomens of several women. My hands gently felt many babies, some alive, many motionless.

Amniotic fluid is needed around the baby for survival. If the mother faces dehydration, her body will utilize any fluids it can find to save her, even the fluids around her baby. This can easily lead to fetal death.

One of every ten women I laid hands on had already experienced a fetal death, probably from the earthquake trauma. Post-traumatic stress and family death, falling debris or internal injuries to the mothers most likely caused the demise of their babies. Other mothers now faced the deliveries of their babies without hospitals and possibly without a health care provider.

During the prenatal exams, many women shared their experience about being "buried alive" amidst concrete and debris. They disclosed the loss of other children, husbands, and family members. Many Haitians now feared being buried alive. Many refused to enter any buildings that were still standing due to recurrent aftershocks and fear of the falling buildings. Our clinic remained outside; our supplies inside.

It is believed that there were over 37,000 pregnant women in Haiti at the time of the earthquake. Many delivered their babies into the hands of a willing friend or a helpful Samaritan. Many died. One mother in the clinic asked, "Where will I go to have my baby? I have nothing—no food, no diapers, no place to go."

This request was typical. We could only assess the mothers' needs and do our best to minimize their ailments. I knew my time in Haiti was not long enough to do more, so I needed to develop a plan for these desperate mothers.

In my broken French, I asked any local health care provider living in the tent city to come and work with our team. Within minutes, a woman approached me. Julienne was a midwife. I invited her to work with me. I learned that Julienne had lost her husband and children in the earthquake. She lived in a nearby tent and invited me to her make-shift home.

Julienne's tent was a white tarp lined from side to side with blankets. She showed me her birth box of supplies that she took for any births she attended. It was empty. Yesterday, she had delivered five babies in the tent city of Carrefour. Today she was out of supplies.

We worked together until we could no longer see women in the waning dusk. Both of us were exhausted and needed rest, but we pressed on. We developed plans and strategies with each client to aid them in birth. We packaged birth supplies for each mother to use, and instructed each of them to call for Julienne when their time came.

I filled Julienne's box with instruments, medicine, towels, gloves and cord clamps. Our team packed to leave for the day, and as I mounted the truck, I turned back and saw Julienne. She was on top of the clinic building. Her hands were lifted high and her eyes looked to the heavens. She was praying. She then reached out, wrapped in her own sorrow and need, and blessed the entire tent city.

"I took you from the ends of the earth, from it farthest corner I called you. I said, 'You are my servant,' I have chosen you and have not rejected you." Isaiah 41:9

There is an ongoing need for strategic health care focus to continue in Haiti. This is a long-term effort for a minimum of ten years until homes, hospitals, and Port au Prince is rebuilt. The future health care concern encompasses public health and the spread of disease. The devastation escalates as the reality of homelessness settles in on thousands of survivors. Homelessness is a minor obstacle for those who remain in Haiti when compared to the greater obstacles yet to come. Surviving infection from bone-crushing wounds, lack of proper sanitation, shortage of clean water, and starvation are on the immediate horizon for many.

The overall impression of the current health care situation in Haiti is grave. The lack of running water to wash hands and wounds, places to urinate and the close temporary housing situation are poised to invite infectious disease to spread throughout a community, causing greater death than the Haitians have already seen.

Historically, infectious diseases such as tuberculosis, Hepatitis, typhoid and cholera will grasp the young, the weak, and those who have already suffered the trauma of this recent earthquake. The death toll rises.

May God bless His people in Haiti and cause a revival to fall upon them in their time of need. This outreach founded in the wonderful giving of our nation. Thank God for Americans, may God bless America.

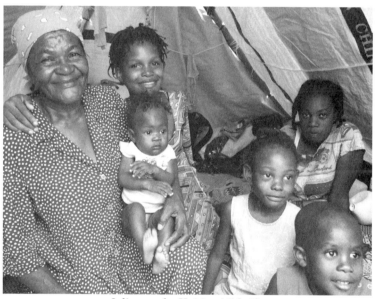

Julienne, the Haitian Midwife.

Seige

As I walked through the beaten sand of a West African city, my feet felt the warmth of the sand around my toes. The city was crowded with people, and I was jostled as I looked for my favorite vendor. A towering Black African woman, who made her daily wage by mixing a cake paste, was sitting on the same corner I always found her. She fried the paste, dropping it by the spoonful, into a tin bowl filled with hot oil. The bowl balanced precariously over a charcoal fire. Her children sat quietly at her side, watching me—the "white woman." Their big brown eyes fixated on my white freckled arms. One reached out to touch me but cowered back when my eyes met his. I smiled. Their clothes were torn, dirty and barely covered their small lean bodies. A close-knit family caught in the cycle of poverty in West Africa.

An entrepreneur of sorts, this woman daily purchased her needed supplies of oil, eggs, flour and charcoal. She always positioned herself on the corner of the market to lure hungry shoppers like me. My mission was not to shop, but to purchase her fresh cakes as a late-night snack.

We were not strangers. I had met her several years prior when she presented to the clinic where I worked. She was in labor, and I delivered her last baby.

I called the fried cakes donuts, and the little family laughed. The woman gently wrapped about ten in a paper for me. The fee was 50 ouguiya. Conveniently, I never had change and always paid her 100 ouguiya, which equaled about 35 cents in U.S. dollars. The donuts were hot and freshly doused with sugar, so I tucked them inside my backpack and headed to the clinic.

Spring was ending and summer's heat climbed to over forty degrees Celsius. The sand was so hot we could not walk without shoes. Even if the sand was cool, I would not walk barefoot. Trash and debris littered the streets. The sand was black from the exhaust of cars, droppings of donkeys, goats, mutton, and human excrement. I rarely walked beside buildings anymore because people squatted near them to defecate or urinate. The government had no plan for proper sanitation.

I had worked in Mauritania for over four years, and I was accustomed to the filth. I didn't approve of it; I was just used to it. I had learned how to deal with it, or in some cases, to just walk around it. My mission in public health was to change childbirth in the country; not improve street cleanliness.

Over the past few years, I had learned many of the obstacles women faced in childbirth. I had hoped to somehow impact one life at a time; to make a difference. Entering the clinic compound, my eyes searched the ground. I tried to avoid any medical waste that may be lurking, ready to snag my toes. Often I found syringes buried in the sand. This frustrated me—medical waste on the compound. Today was different; no trash on the ground.

A smile started to cross my face. As I approached the clinic doors, I viewed the signs I had hung months before. Barely hanging, the signs gathered blowing sand, but still conveyed their message.

"Dispose of Medical Waste Properly." The handmade posters, made by American nursing students, showed pictures of a hand placing syringes, needles, blood-soaked items and medical waste in a red trash can. After several teaching sessions, we all hoped that the local health care providers understood the importance of properly disposing of needles and waste. The signs made an impact.

Nine months had passed since Ramadan had ended, ushering in a high birth season in the government-run maternity centers. The entry to the delivery area was full of families sitting on the ground and huddled together atop the tile concrete benches. I stopped to greet each family, nod at the men, and shake the hands of each woman. I knew it was unusual for them to see a "white woman." I was obviously a foreigner. I was hopeful that my greeting would lessen any fear. Even in an urgent situation, I knew that a proper greeting was a priority.

"Salam-a-lakin," I said.

"Lakin salam," they replied. They smiled and nodded. They believed that when a foreigner came to the clinic, it was a sign of authority and excellence. I was always amazed at how they welcomed me. They asked me if I felt safe in their country.

The "sage femme's quarters" or midwives' room was a small 9x9 place with wall to wall mats placed strategically for resting. This day, it was empty. I quickly reached into my backpack for my supplies, covered my scrubs with a lab coat and proceeded to the delivery area. Three 4x4 stainless steel tables were used for deliveries. Women walked to these tables prior to delivery, stepped up on to the table, somehow fitted their legs back onto the small area, and pushed their babies out.

All three tables were full. I glanced past a curtain separating the area from another very small room and saw three other women in labor. We were going to have a busy night.

The only sink for the entire center was located in the delivery room against the far wall. It was full of dirty instruments and bedpans. I quickly reached over to wash my hands and prepare for deliveries. Currently, only one other midwife worked at the center. It was obvious she needed help. I turned the faucet, but nothing happened. There was no running water—again.

I immediately called out to the families in the waiting area, "Find our guard and ask him to get us water." Then I reached for my gloves, just as I heard the moans of a mother change to grunts.

The other midwife, Fatimah, was an apprentice and in her first year of training in the birth theatre. She had already delivered over 100 babies, but was still considered inexperienced. Each apprentice trained for at least three years in the capital city, then returned to their villages to be the local health care provider and midwife. After three years of apprenticeship, they gained the title of "Sage Femme," which means "wise woman" in their national language of French.

Fatimah triaged some of the laboring women and asked me to check the woman on the delivery table who was grunting and rocking herself back and forth. She was in full labor and appeared to be pushing.

"Is this your first baby?" I asked. "Is there only one? When were you due?"

No answers, she did not speak French.

Fatimah talked to her in Pular then answered me in French. Unfortunately, the woman had not received any prenatal care. She just came to the clinic, already in labor.

Using my Doppler, I listened to the baby whose heart rate was around 120, fabulous. I examined the mother. She indeed was fully dilated and pushing. But that was not a head presenting. It was the butt and the feet. Sweat beaded on my brow while adrenaline rushed through my body. I had never delivered a breech baby and my only assistant was an apprentice.

I called out to Fatimah, "Le bébé est par le siège."

She looked at me with puzzled eyes and said, "Ce que vous a fait dit." (In English, "What did you say?")

I repeated my words twice, and she still looked at me, puzzled. I pointed to my own booty and said, "Siege."

Fatimah stared at me, motionless. So I reached over, grabbed her bottom and said, "Le bébé est par le siège." Her eyes widened.

Obviously, my Midwestern twang and French were not very clear to her smooth African/Arabic French. Within a few minutes, as the mother continued to push, I gently swiped the babies' hips, reducing the feet. The feet and legs began to emerge.

Panic swept Fatimah's face as she raised her hands to her face and covered her eyes with her veil. She ran out of the room. Although my thoughts went crazy, I turned to the mother and locked my eyes with hers. I smiled, nodded and very calmly encouraged her to keep pushing.

The baby's kicking legs and hips gently emerged. I was thrilled that he kicked; believing this to be a sign of normalcy and that the cord was not crushed between his body and the mother's pelvis. Another push and his body began to slide forward. His chest and back appeared, so I reached deep into my backpack to grab a clean towel. Sterile technique was now the least of my concerns. I was alone in the delivery room with three women in labor and a breech presentation.

"Lord Jesus, help me," I prayed.

Wrapping the body with my towel, I waited for the head to be born. I watched his black curly hairline peek through as his neck appeared, but the head did not advance. His kicking ceased. The umbilical cord went white and pulsing ceased. Time was now of the essence. This baby needed to be born, now—all of him.

Where was Fatima?

My hands reached around the baby's body, grasping over the towel I had draped to shield him from the cooler air. Gently I extended his body, then flexed and rotated while encouraging the mother to push. Both arms and shoulder delivered, but his head remained. It emerged slightly, and then quickly retreated into the womb. The head would not pass beneath the pelvic bones of the mother.

I now held his motionless body in my hands. His head was wedged tightly in the grasp of his mother's body. "Please, God. Give me guidance, grace and supernatural courage." I feared the worst—death.

Another contraction mounted, and while I firmly gazed into the eyes of the would-be mother, I stated "Poussée mamma, beaucoup poussée."

She began with all her might to push as I slipped my fingers into the mouth of the baby. I pulled down on his mouth to flex his head and lowered his body to aid in the flexion, then lifted it to a neutral position as it finally gave and passed the outlet. He was born. Praise be to God!

He gasped, but seemed only to make the motion without taking a breath. I began drying his body and talking to him as I lifted his limp core to his mother's abdomen. "Come on, baby. You can do it. Come on, baby."

He whimpered. His heart rate was pounding; his breathing was weak. He was not moving.

"Come on, baby. You can do it." I continued to speak to him, and then he began to cry. Behind me, someone cheered and clapped. I looked up to see Fatimah standing behind me, with a smile covering her face. She had hurried out to get another midwife to help with the breech delivery. They had returned to the clinic just as the baby was born.

I smiled and gave thanks to God. The women surrounded us and prayed to Allah, their God, to deliver them as well with a healthy baby. They smiled, nodded and gave the thumbs up signal as Africans do when they are happy.

"Is any one of you in trouble? He should pray. Is anyone happy? Let him sing songs of praise." James 5:13

Reflecting on this birth, I realized that no matter how much education I have, I am constantly learning and growing. In this particular situation, I was the highest educated health care provider in the area, holding two postgraduate degrees. I was also the health care provider who lacked experience with breech deliveries. I learned the "how to do it" version by reading textbooks during my midwifery training. However, except on video, I had never seen a breech birth. Unfortunately, I was still the highest skilled practitioner available on this given day. This mother had no other options.

Since that day, I have delivered several breech babies, all in Africa. By the grace of God, they have all lived. I am not sure I will ever carry this experience back home to the U.S., due to practice restrictions. The physicians I currently work with do not allow breech deliveries outside of the hospital, and my practice is in a birth center.

Sadly, women throughout the continent of Africa are faced with the same challenges in birth and their outcomes are not always so positive. About 3-4 percent of all women globally present in labor with a breech presentation. I have met several midwives and physicians across the globe who are experienced with breech deliveries. However, there are very few in America.

Furthermore, women in many developing countries do not have the option to go to the local hospital and have a cesarean section. The best option is to have a trained birth attendant available to safely deliver their baby. According to the World Health Organization, one out of every five babies in Africa will die during the first year of life. This alarming statistic is why they promote the policy for every woman to have a trained birth attendant present when they deliver.

I would never recommend that midwives or physicians purchase an airline ticket, go to Africa and learn the "How to Catch a Breech Baby" process. However, I do highly encourage them to get that plane ticket and learn the mechanics of birth from other midwives and physicians. The skills these practitioners have in utilizing their assessment of each client and their gifted hands at a birth are remarkable. They can deliver breech babies, twins and difficult presentations because they have to.

Learning breech delivery is very difficult in the U.S., because most are delivered by cesarean section. In America, women have more health care providers to access, but fewer birth options and choices when they go into labor with a breech presentation. The medical-legal forces of our litigious society prohibits women from choosing vaginal breech birth as an option.

In addition, it is very hard to find a practitioner who feels confident and is willing to perform a vaginal breech delivery. Many women are using the secrecy of their homes to vaginally deliver their breech babies. The providers they find to aid in the delivery of their babies are also working in secrecy. Rarely do providers advertise they perform breech deliveries because they do not want to face the unwanted negative press regarding the risks. The negativity surrounding breech deliveries is so focused on the bad outcome that most providers fear advertisement would "close their doors" of opportunity for women who desire vaginal breech birth.

The most important consideration prior to a breech birth is turning the baby. The only way to know if your baby is breech is by going to your regularly scheduled prenatal appointments and having your provider palpate your abdomen. If there is ever a doubt as to what is the presenting part of the baby, such as the head or buttocks, then an ultrasound can be ordered to confirm it.

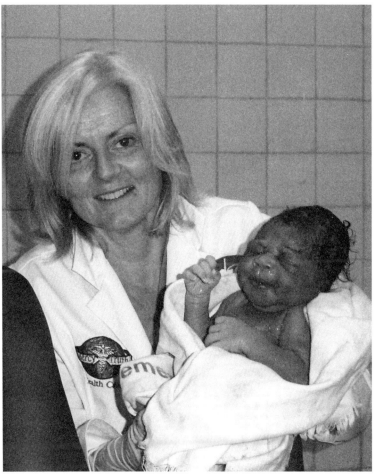

Cathy holding breech baby after birth.

They All Rallied

The doors flew open, clanging the metal frames against the cement walls. The sound penetrated the hall like an explosion from a blown tire. Everyone in the obstetrical wards halted their tasks to turn and stare at the commotion.

A man burst through the entry, carrying the body of his wife. Long, dark fabrics covered every inch of her body except her face. Her eyes were closed and sunken; her skin pale and placid.

I was working at a National Hospital in Africa, serving as a health care consultant and midwife in labor and delivery. At the time, it was the only hospital in the entire country. People traveled for miles in the desert to seek healthcare. The hospital stood as a beacon of hope to many facing disease, birth defects and death itself.

This hospital accepted clients from outlying clinics who were having difficulties giving birth or who had given birth but had complications. No official transfer policy or emergency system was in place. When women required health care that they could not receive in another setting such as their own home or a government-based clinic, they would come to the hospital.

"Salem-a lakin," I said while I motioned for the man to lay his wife down on a bed. I approached her side. She was limp and motionless. Her eyes closed. I could not tell if she was breathing;

she looked dead. My hand searched beneath her veil and palpated her neck. I felt for a pulse. I also reached for my stethoscope, and removed her veil so I could listen for heart sounds. As I leaned in closer to place my stethoscope on her chest, her dark, sunken eyes opened.

I jumped back as if I had seen a ghost. She seemed so vacant, but obviously alive. Her dry cracked lips moved, but no sound came out. I began my rapid assessment. Scanning her veil-draped body, I noted that she had been bleeding. The lower segment of her veil was saturated with blood. The mucous membranes surrounding her teeth were white and the conjunctiva of her eyes lacked any color at all. Her pulse was very faint and thready. She was alive, but barely.

I looked at her husband and asked him in my best broken Arabic, "What happened? What is the problem?"

He did not respond, but stood next to her as if nothing else existed in the world. He seemed to be in a state of shock.

A woman who followed them in approached and spoke to me in French, "My sister is sick." Tears dropped from her face. "Her husband returned after a long journey and found her like this, so he asked me to care for her but she was too sick; too weak."

She stopped to blow her nose and then began again, "My sister told me she thought she was pregnant and close to birth. She didn't want her husband to leave on his journey, but he went anyway."

A long silence hung in the air as the sister turned and scowled at the sullen man.

"Okay" I added, "go on." I needed to know what had happened.

Her voice softened and she continued, while leaning in to comfort her sister, "It is customary for women preparing to give birth to return to their mother's home so that they can be cared for. Unfortunately, our mother is not alive." She sighed, while gently stroking her sister's forehead. "My sister started to have pain and bleed, but there was no baby, just blood. It has been several days since this has happened."

While the sister talked, my eyes scanned the woman's body. She had no rounded abdomen, as a pregnant woman would display. Her abdomen was sunken and concave to her umbilicus; she was thin and frail. I palpated the uterus; firm just below the umbilicus. Using my Doppler, I heard no fetal heart tones.

Quickly I grabbed my backpack to retrieve my Hemo-que, a rapid hemoglobin analyzer. I pricked her finger and squeezed, hoping to check her quick hemoglobin. By presentation alone, she seemed anemic. No blood came from her finger, just the yellow twinge of serum.

That is so weird, I thought, as I repricked her finger and found the same result. Her head turned toward mine and her eyes fixed on me. I milked her finger, hoping to get just one drop of blood. Finally, a drop fell onto the cuvette and I immediately placed it in the analyzer. The reading was 0.9gm/dl.

My mind went into denial, *How can this woman be alive with such a low hemoglobin? That can't be possible.*

Normal hemoglobin is between 12-14gm/dl for women and her level was 0.9gm/dl. I recalibrated my machine, hoping that was the problem. It calibrated perfectly, so I reinserted her cuvette. The result was unchanged. I needed to move quickly or this mother would die.

I summoned the nurses to get an immediate lab on this woman and initiate an IV. We needed to confirm my hemoglobin results. I asked for one of the surgeons to come stat to the Obstetrical unit. Everyone responded so efficiently. Her IV slid in easily which was a miracle in itself. The IV now flowed wide open; a life-line for this woman.

"Can we give her a blood transfusion?" I asked the nurses, knowing there was no blood bank or volume expanders or plasma in the entire hospital. The nurses nodded in affirmation and disappeared.

"Come back," I shouted at them. "Come back." I could not understand why they had left the room; we had a life to save.

The doors burst open again. This time it was the lab technician, carrying the results. "Surely there must be a mistake," he said. "The results are very low."

My worst fear was confirmed; this woman was bleeding to death. *Where were the nurses and the surgeon?*

Just then, I heard voices and movement behind me. The nurses returned to the ward and led a group of about twenty people into the room.

"Stop! I can't have all these people here. Please help me with this woman," I pleaded.

One of the nurses grabbed my hand and said, "They have come to give blood." She paused briefly and repeated, "They have all rallied and come to give blood to this woman, to help her."

I scanned the faces of the people. Mothers, sisters, fathers, brothers, family members, friends and people who wanted to help me and help this woman. I soon learned that the nurses went to the hospital reception area and asked for anyone willing to give blood to come to the unit. They explained that I had made a request for blood and they needed to find willing donors right now. These people all came, wanting to help save the life of someone they did not know. Some cried. Others were silent.

The lab technician encouraged all of the willing donors to come to the lab. Every potential donor was tested for HIV, using a rapid identification test to determine his or her blood type. If they were HIV negative and had the same blood type, they could give blood.

Five people were selected, and stood in the hall waiting to help the woman. Each donor prepped for the procedure by diligently washing their hands and arms with soap and water. The first donor lay down on a cart next to the woman. A large needle was inserted into the donor's arm, and then tubing used gravity to drain the blood from the donor directly to the woman.

One donor on the table and four others waited in place. But the woman died before she could receive one drop of blood.

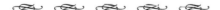

The World Health Organization (WHO) and United Nations, are working together to improve maternal health worldwide. Hemorrhage or bleeding because of childbirth remains one of the leading global causes of maternal death.

Millennium Development Goals 5: improve maternal health

Target 5.A. Reduce by three quarters, between 1990 and 2015, the maternal mortality ratio

Up to 358,000 women die each year in pregnancy and childbirth. Most of them die because they have no access to skilled routine and emergency care. Since 1990, some countries in Asia and Northern Africa have more than halved maternal mortality. Sub-Saharan Africa has also seen progress. Unlike in the developed world where a woman's lifetime risk of dying during or following pregnancy is 1 in 4,300, the risk of maternal death in undeveloped countries is one in thirty-one. Increasing numbers of women are now seeking care in health facilities; therefore, it is important to ensure that the quality of care provided is optimal. "Making Pregnancy Safer," a campaign as part of the World Health Organization, focuses its activities on seventy-five priority countries in which 97 percent of all maternal deaths worldwide occur. Half of the countries are located in the African Region.

The Bible tells a story of a woman who had been bleeding for years, **"Just then, a woman who had been subject to bleeding for twelve years came up behind him and touched the edge of his cloak" (Matt. 9:20).**

This woman had tried all the resources available to her to stop the bleeding. Her faith led her to seek out the healer, Jesus, whom she heard about from friends. Her healing that day was a result of her faith.

We can also walk in the same faith, knowledge and power to come against these obstacles for women by being their voice and taking action to impact their lives. Today I am the voice of the woman in this chapter, to tell her story so that others will not succumb to the same fate. I believe that God is using me to be her voice and invite all readers to join in the fight to improve maternal health in the world.

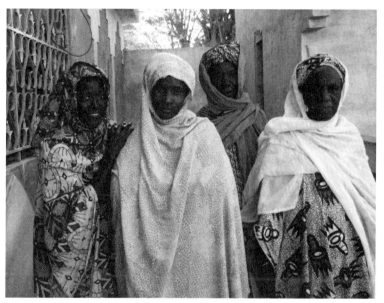

Mauritanian Midwives, my friends and colleagues.

Hello Means Goodbye

The young mother looked vacantly into my eyes while beads of sweat dripped from her brow. Strong contractions grasped her tiny womb every two to three minutes. They seemed to mount one after the other. She made no sound. Tension showed on her face as the contractions surged to their height. It was well over forty degrees Celsius outside and she had walked several miles to the clinic. She was exhausted, but her small belly rose, rounded and surged forward with each contraction.

Her tiny frame barely looked pregnant. She measured small for active labor, about thirty-two centimeters. I placed my hands on her belly to assess the baby's size, position and presentation. The shape was not normal. My hands gently palpated the baby. It felt odd. My hands became my eyes and they saw a different shape, not symmetrical and very awkward. My hands smoothly surfed the contractions and contour of her abdomen.

What am I feeling I wondered as I continued my exam, *where is the baby's head?*

Several years ago while working in the same clinic, I learned a valuable lesson. The midwives taught me to value my hands and consider them as my eyes. I learned that the actual "laying on of hands" could tell me so much. My hands could bridge the barriers of language, culture and religion and give midwife guidance. These talented midwives demonstrated how their hands could determine the size, position and presentation of a baby so accurately one would have thought they had a secret ultrasound in another room. They took the time to guide and train my hands with theirs. I worked with these midwives for weeks, training my hands to be my eyes.

Gently palpating every aspect of the young mother's abdomen, I envisioned the baby. The mother had minimal fluid, making it easy to identify different aspects of the baby's anatomy. My hands felt the prominence of the backbone, the hips, and the shoulders. I followed the backbone down to the head. Yes, it was presenting low in the pelvis.

But there was more. I followed the back bone up and as it rounded the buttocks, I felt another firm baseball form. Grasping this ball, my hands gently caressed it and followed it along another firm backbone. Two babies lived in this small womb, and they were about ready to be born.

Adrenaline rushed through my body as I turned to my African colleague and said, "Il y a deux bébés" (there are two babies) I knew we were not prepared to have twins, especially early twins.

Another contraction tightened the belly of this young African woman, and she instinctively bared down to push. She was twenty-four years old and about to give birth to her very first baby, one she had prayed for since her marriage. I prepared for the ultimate birth of the twins. Gathering supplies, I hoped my hands were wrong about the size of these babies, but my instinct told me she was about to give birth to premature twins. I wanted so badly to call for a neonatal team, but there was none.

Our clinic, located in West Africa, provided labor and delivery services to about 4,000 families annually. It was always busy. The single delivery room had three exam tables lined up side by side to serve as delivery tables. There was one sink and one trash can in the room. Each mother who entered could watch, hear and smell another woman giving birth. The constant unique smell of birth hovered in the air.

Another contraction surged over the body of this mother-to-be. The tiny head of the baby emerged. Hungry to be born, she looked around. Her eyes blinked and quickly closed as light shone upon them for the first time. Her head was about the size of a large tangerine; her body just over sixteen inches long. She gently slid out of her mother. Her tiny hand reached up and grasped my finger. Like a rock climber on his lifeline, she reached for life and hung on. She wanted to live. She cried and breathed in life, then vigorously moved her arms and legs. She weighed one pound, eight ounces.

I handed her over to my assistant as another contraction mounted. Within minutes, the bottom of baby number two emerged. Gently, she was born. She whimpered, but was not vigorous. I rubbed her back and whispered to her, "Come on, baby girl, you can do it. You can live today."

What was I thinking? We had no neonatal team, no oxygen, no nurses, no ventilators or medications. I had no resuscitation equipment at this clinic except suction and myself, of course. I had no surfactant. I had no IV. I had only my "what if" thoughts.

What if these tiny girls live? Why can't they?

What if they are just small for their age? There is that possibility.

What if a miracle happens today and they... live?

My eyes scanned their tiny bodies as I continued to massage them. It was obvious they were born too soon. Thin, wrinkly skin covered their lean bodies. They lacked vernix—the white cheesy coating often seen on late pre-term and full-term babies. They had fine downy hair.

Born too early, but I wanted to believe in a miracle. I wanted so badly for these babies to live. "Please God; help me help these tiny babies. Please, God."

I dried the second baby and encouraged her to take in breath. She tried, but her cry seemed much weaker. Gently, I rubbed her back, then her feet. "Come on baby, live for your momma."

I looked at my assistant, as she held the first girl who was now barely breathing. Deep down I knew there was nothing I could do to aid these babies today. Nevertheless, how could we not try? I wanted the new mother to hold her girls with joy; not sorrow.

How can "Hello" mean "Goodbye?"

The tiny babies' cries for life grew weaker and their color began to change. Carefully I laid the babies together and gently swaddled them next to each other. I offered the babies to the mother, but she refused to hold them. It was as if she knew what was happening.

I understood her feelings, but I could not just lay them aside. Together, they were bundled; together they would die. I held them closely now and sang to them, "Jesus loves the little children, all the children of the world."

The baby girls snuggled with each other as their color darkened and they no longer cried. Their rose bud lips opened and gasped for air, but their weak bodies could no longer take in the breath. Their air-hungry breathing slowed. Within minutes, they no longer moved. Her babies died in my arms as the mother watched. I could do nothing for them.

If only we were in the U.S., we could help these babies.

If only they were a little older.

If only I had supplies.

If only this clinic were more equipped, but this is the highest level of care in the country.

All of my "if only" thoughts were in vain. None would make a difference today. I could do nothing more but hold their bodies and sing, "Jesus loves the little children, all the children of the world."

Not long after I returned home, a friend of mine went into early labor. She was also pregnant with twins. Her babies were only twenty-seven weeks gestation. The babies I delivered in Africa were slightly older, estimated at about thirty weeks gestation.

Both women were pregnant with twins and each woman so desperately wanted to be a mother. One mother lived in an affluent country, where myriads of specialists surrounded her and her babies. One lived in Africa, where maternal child health disparities soar where no team of specialists gathers to help babies live.

One mother held her babies; one mother did not.

My friend's babies lived. Today her boys are healthy, attend school and suffer no ill effects from being born to soon, because they were given an opportunity.

More babies are born each day in Africa than any other continent of the world. Sadly, more babies also die each day in Africa than in any other continent of the world. Mothers in Africa desire to hold and love their babies just like the mothers in America. Unfortunately, they are not born with the equal opportunity for life.

I believe God has a distinct purpose in revealing this story.

Les Amis de Naissance, which means "friends of birth", is a non-profit organization focused on improving maternal-child health globally. Currently they are working on projects to aid international midwives in many countries. Perhaps someone who reads this story will collaborate with Les Amis de Naissance to change and impact birth for all mothers.

The Bible reveals to us in Romans 8:28 that **"All things work together for the good of those who love him and have been called according to his purpose."**

All things; even the living and dying of tiny babies.

About The Author

Catherine Gordon, "Cathy" is an authority on midwifery and birth centers, leading the creation of two birth centers in the greater Kansas City, delivering babies in over nine different countries, and a mother of four herself. Cathy founded Mercy &Truth Medical Missions in 1994 and served as CEO for fifteen years. Currently she is the CEO and co-founder of the NEW BIRTH COMPANY in Overland Park and serves as faculty with Mid-America Nazarene University. She speaks, teaches and writes on a variety of issues effecting freestanding birth centers, maternal child disparities, and global health. Her latest endeavor is the inception of a new non-profit called Les Amis de Naissance, which means "The friends of birth." This organization will strive to combat birth disparity and enable "Incredible BIRTH Days" for all women in all nations.

Cathy earned her B.S. and M.S. in Science from the University of Kansas. She is a certified nurse midwife and board certified family nurse practitioner and has been the recipient of a variety of awards including most recently a "Kansas City Shining Star Award" from the Maternal Child Health Coalition and International volunteer service proclamation from Kansas City's Mayor, Mark Funkhouser.

Whether you want to purchase bulk copies of *All Babies Are Born* or buy another book for a friend, get it now at: www.imprbooks.com.

If you have a book that you would like to publish, contact Terry Whalin, Publisher, at Intermedia Publishing Group, (623) 337-8710 or email: twhalin@intermediapub.com or use the contact form at: www.intermediapub.com.

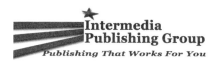